PHYSICAL EXAMINATION
of the
HEART AND CIRCULATION

Second Edition

JOSEPH K. PERLOFF, M.D.

Streisand/American Heart Association Professor
of Medicine and Pediatrics,
UCLA School of Medicine, Los Angeles, California

1990

W. B. SAUNDERS COMPANY
Harcourt Brace Jovanovich, Inc.

Philadelphia, London, Toronto, Montreal, Sydney, Tokyo

W. B. SAUNDERS COMPANY
Harcourt Brace Jovanovich, Inc.

The Curtis Center
Independence Square West
Philadelphia, PA 19106

Library of Congress Cataloging-in-Publication Data

Perloff, Joseph K., 1924–

Physical examination of the heart and circulation / by
  Joseph K. Perloff.—2nd ed.
    p.   cm.
Includes bibliographies and index.

ISBN 0–7216–7189–6

1. Heart—Examination.   2. Cardiovascular system—
  Examination.   3. Physical diagnosis.   I. Title.
  [DNLM: 1. Blood Circulation.   2. Heart Diseases—
  diagnosis.   3. Physical Examination.   WG 141 P451p]
RC683.P397 1990   616.1′0754—dc20   89–10204
DNLM/DLC

Listed below are the latest translations of this book together with the name of
the publisher:

Japanese—*first edition*—HBJ Japan, Inc.

Portuguese—*first edition*—Publ. Internacionals Revinter Ltda., Rus do Matoso,
                195-D Tijuca CEP 20270, Rio de Janeiro, Brazil

Spanish—*first edition*—Panamericana, C.C. 70, Sucursal 53, Buenos Aires,
                Argentino

Acquisition Editor: William Lamsback
Production Manager: Frank Polizzano
Manuscript Editor: Donna Walker
Illustration Coordinator: Joan Sinclair
Indexer: George Vilk

COVER ILLUSTRATION: Palpation of the
radial pulse as illustrated in *The Yellow
Emperor's Classic of Internal Medicine*,
the oldest medical book still extant.

Physical Examination of the Heart and Circulation   ISBN 0–7216–7189–6

Last digit is the print number: 9   8   7   6   5   4   3   2   1

To the memory of
PAUL HAMILTON WOOD
*from whom I learned
the physical examination
of the heart and
circulation.*

And to those whom I have taught
and will teach, "For you have I prepared
this book on physical diagnoses. In its
preparation I have endeavored to be concise,
yet clear and comprehensive. Its name
indicates its object; viz. to give you, in a
compact form, a complete view of what
are technically called the physical signs."

HENRY I. BOWDITCH
The Young Stethoscopist, 1848

ACKNOWLEDGMENTS

My largest debt is to the late Dr. Paul H. Wood, from whom, more than anyone, I learned the physical examination of the heart and circulation. To the Fulbright Fellowship Program and the Institute for International Education I shall always be grateful for making it possible for me to spend a formative year working closely with Dr. Wood and his colleagues at the Institute of Cardiology and the National Heart Hospital in London.

It has become commonplace to pay respect to the students, house staff, and fellows with whom one works, but the truth of the matter is that these intelligent, enthusiastic, receptive, yet critical young people provided the stimulus that gave necessary impetus to my efforts.

It is a pleasure to acknowledge the Streisand/American Heart Association Professorship Endowment, the Rosalind W. Alcott Endowment, and the National Heart, Lung and Blood Institute Training Grant No. HL7412 to the Division of Cardiology, Department of Medicine, University of California, Los Angeles.

I am especially grateful to my wife Marjorie for having contributed so much to a lively intellectual environment that put a premium on scholarly achievement. Her integrity has furnished me with a virtually unattainable standard and made her my most effective critic. Her praise, not given lightly, was all the more gratifying. Her tolerance of my idiosyncrasies was not the least of her many virtues.

JOSEPH K. PERLOFF, M.D.

PREFACE

> The methods of examination, as commonly taught
> and pursued, are often assumed to be so complete
> that no further progress can be made unless by the
> employment of some new mechanical means—so
> that it is asserted there can be no further advances
> in the examination of the patient by the unaided
> senses.
>
> *Sir James Mackenzie, 1916**

Sophisticated laboratory methods provide contemporary clinicians with stunning diagnostic insights but, in so doing, risk de-emphasizing the bedside examination upon which previous generations were much more dependent and therefore much more adept. Lest we feel that these concerns are peculiar to our time, recall the preface to Sir James Mackenzie's *Principles of Diagnosis and Treatment in Heart Affections* (1916), in which he wrote, "A great deal of our recent knowledge of heart conditions has been attained by the use of such mechanical aids as the polygraph and the electrocardiograph. . . . It has been a constant endeavor on my part to recognize the different conditions which these instruments have revealed by employing the ordinary bedside methods of examination, and I am concerned mainly with them in this book." My objective in writing a book on the physical examination of the heart and circulation is to bring to the reader the results of my own experience in employing ordinary bedside methods of examination. These methods beautifully supplement the remarkable laboratory techniques that have done so much to reveal the meanings and increase the diagnostic value of cardiovascular physical signs.

---

*Mackenzie, J.: Principles of Diagnosis and Treatment in Heart Affections. London, Oxford University Press, 1916.

The original or early descriptions of a host of cardio-vascular physical signs are impossible to improve upon for accuracy and clarity of language. I have liberally drawn from these early descriptions, which not only excite admiration for our predecessors, but, I hope, will also serve to make my book more interesting by bringing the reader closer to a distinguished past.

CONTENTS

INTRODUCTION WITH A BRIEF HISTORICAL SURVEY

Every physician of experience works out . . . a method of examination, and though the methods of different physicians may vary, yet the object is the same in every case, namely, to get as much knowledge as possible. . . .[1]

SIR JAMES MACKENZIE

The physical examination of the cardiovascular system deals with the heart and circulation per se, with the chest and abdomen, and with the physical signs of coexisting noncardiac diseases that modify or shed light on cardiovascular disorders. Examination of the heart and circulation includes (1) physical appearance (sometimes called inspection), (2) the arterial pulse, (3) the jugular and peripheral veins, (4) the location and movements of the heart—percussion, palpation, and observation of the precordium, and (5) auscultation. Examination of the chest and abdomen frequently reveals signs secondary to or associated with cardiac or vascular disorders. In infants, children, and young adults, diseases of the heart are likely to occur in otherwise normal patients. With advancing age, coexisting noncardiac diseases modify the cardiovascular physical signs.

Systematic assessment of each physical sign sets the stage for a synthesis of information based upon these signs. It is axiomatic that emphasis should focus on the relationship of the parts to the whole, a relationship that ideally results in a harmonious picture devoid of contradictions, not an assembly of loosely related observations. Maximum information should be extracted from each physical sign while relating information from one sign to that of another.

No organ system lends itself better to a close association between signs, structure, and function than the heart and circulation. Laboratory characterization of cardiovascular anatomy and physiology has validated these signs, which in turn permit remarkably precise pathophysiologic inferences to be drawn from them. Excitement, satisfaction, and a feeling of confidence and security are experienced when an abundance of accurate, practical information is assembled with the unaided senses apart from a stethoscope, a sphygmomanometer, an ophthalmoscope, and a pocket flashlight.

My purpose is to describe physical signs and how they are best elicited. I will deal with mechanisms chiefly when so doing serves this end. Emphasis is placed upon the physical *examination* rather than physical diagnosis.

The fabric of the modern cardiovascular physical examination is woven from threads of the past. Franciscus de le Boe Sylvius, Chair of Medicine at the University of Leiden, was one of the most celebrated clinical teachers of the seventeenth century and was the first champion of bedside teaching in medical education. He wrote that he would " . . . lead my students by the hand to the practice of medicine, taking them every day to see patients in the public hospital, that they may hear the patients' symptoms and see their physical findings."[2] Two and one-half centuries later, Harvey Cushing's biography of William Osler began with the dedication: "To medical students in the hope that something of Osler's spirit may be conveyed to those of a generation that has not known him; and particularly to those in America, lest it be forgotten who it was that made it possible for them to work at the bedside in the wards."[3]

All five essential components of the cardiovascular physical examination are rooted in history. Let me touch briefly on each of them.

"The patient's **physical appearance**" was the title of

the introductory paragraph of the chapter "Preliminary Examination of the Patient" in James Mackenzie's *Diseases of the Heart* (1908).[4] "The attempt to appreciate the patient's condition should begin when first he presents himself before us. On his appearance in the consulting-room, his bearing, his gait, the condition of his respiration, the color of his face, any nervous peculiarity in his manner of speech and behavior, and so forth, should be noted. If he is in bed, note the position he assumes, and any change in his color or respiration in response to such exertions as talking or turning over. By habit, one unconsciously notices these things . . . ."

Study of the **arterial pulse** served as the basis for an entire system of diagnostic medicine originating in approximately 2600 B.C. in China with *The Yellow Emperor's Book of Medicine.*[5] *Nei Ching Su Wen* is believed to be the oldest medical book still existing.[5] The book takes the form of a dialogue between the legendary Huang Ti (The Yellow Emperor, 2696–2598 B.C.) and his minister Ch'i Po. The chief means of diagnosis employed in *Nei Ching* is the examination of the pulse. All other methods for determining disease were subsidiary to palpation of the pulse. The state of disease was judged by the volume, strength or weakness, and regularity or interruption of the various beats. The examination was a time-consuming affair, taking hours and involving palpation in nearly a dozen sites while the pulse rate was timed by the physician's respiratory excursions. The patient was examined in the very early morning before the physician took food and before the cares of the day distracted him from full concentration. If the patient was female, her right pulses were palpated first (Fig. 1–1).

Despite the early significance attached to the pulse, its origin in the heart beat was not even remotely considered. It was long in coming before Herophilus, in 344 B.C., recognized that the arterial pulse and cardiac impulse were synchronous. Herophilus used a water clock to count the pulse, made analyses of its rate and rhythm, was influenced by musical theories, and evolved an entire rhythmical pulse lore.[6] In 1700, Sir John Floyer commissioned a well-known English watchmaker to construct a

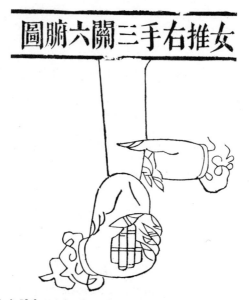

FIGURE 1–1. If the patient was female, her *right* pulses were palpated first, as shown here. If the patient was male, his *left* pulses were examined first. (From The Yellow Emperor's Classic of Internal Medicine, translated by Ilza Veith, University of California Press, Berkeley, 1972, with permission.)

timepiece with a minute hand that permitted accurate determination of the speed of the pulse.[7] In *The Physician's Pulse Watch*, Floyer describes the normal and abnormal arterial pulse, its rate, rhythm, amplitude, forcefulness, and compressibility.[7]

The first recorded description of the **cervical venous pulse** was published in 1728 when Lancisi reported "systolic fluctuation" of the external jugular vein in a patient who at necropsy was found to have tricuspid regurgitation.[8] Rhythmic pulsations of the large veins in the neck were subsequently described by John Hunter in 1794 in his *Treatise on the Blood, Inflammation, and Gun-Shot Wounds.*[9] "The larger veins, near to the heart, have a pulsation which arises from the contraction of the heart preventing the entrance of blood at that time . . . ."[9] Almost a century elapsed before publication by Chauveau and Marey[10] of their classic graphic records of the jugular venous pulse. At the turn of the century, the jugular pulse was shown to have such a striking similarity to the wave forms recorded directly from the right atrium that Carl Wiggers was prompted to write, ". . . it became increasingly more obvious to many physiologists that records of the venous pulse might be of service in the interpretation of dynamic events in the heart."[11] In 1902, James Mackenzie (Fig. 1–2) applied this principle at the bedside in his *Study of the Pulse,*[12] which brought together 20 years of meticulous observation. Mackenzie firmly established the value of the examination of the jugular venous pulse and created a lively interest in its study among clinicians. Paul Wood (Fig. 1–3) did much to rekindle this interest in the 1950's.

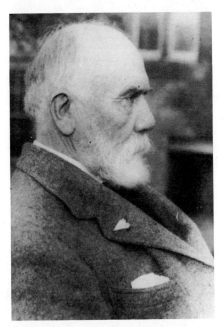

FIGURE 1–2. Sir James Mackenzie (1853–1925). (Courtesy of Katharine E. Donohue, Special Collections Division, Biomedical Library, UCLA Medical Center.)

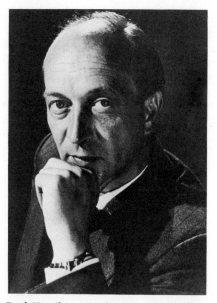

FIGURE 1–3. Paul Hamilton Wood, M.D., OBE (1907–1962). Director of the Institute of Cardiology; Physician to the National Heart Hospital and The Brompton Hospital, London. (Photograph courtesy of Dr. Arthur Selzer, San Francisco.)

The practice of **precordial palpation** was recorded in the Ebers papyrus (1500 B.C.) in a chapter that carried in its title, "Knowledge of the Heart's Movement," which physicians can appreciate by applying their hands or fingers "upon the place of the heart."[13] Systolic movement imparted to the precordium is the most visible evidence of the action of the heart. These movements were familiar to William Harvey early in the seventeenth century. "The heart is erected and rises up to a point so that at this time it strikes against the breast and is felt externally."[14] In 1857, Chauveau confirmed Harvey's contention that precordial movement seen when the heart strikes against the breast resulted from ventricular contraction. Validation awaited Chauveau's animal experiments done in collaboration with Marey, in which an external apex beat was correlated with intracardiac pressure pulses recorded via a catheter.[15]

Leopold Auenbrugger, in his father's inn, witnessed the practice of **percussion** of wine barrels to determine the level of their fluid contents. It later occurred to Auenbrugger that the same technique might be applied to the examination of the human thorax. In 1761, "a kindly and unassuming junior physician at the Vienna Hospital" published his "new invention—inventum novum—for diagnosing thoracic disease by chest percussion."[16] Joseph Skoda hailed the discovery as "the beginning of modern diagnosis," but Auenbrugger's epochal work lay virtually dormant until Corvisart, physician to Napoleon, published an elaborately annotated 480-page French edition of Auenbrugger's unpretentious 95-page book, a step that set the stage for Laënnec's *A Treatise on Diseases of the Chest* (1821).[17]

Auscultation by applying the ear directly to the chest was an established practice in ancient medicine. Hippocratic writings circa 400 B.C. described the "succussion splash" of hydropneumothorax. However, there is no record of precordial auscultation until William Harvey, in 1616, referred to the heartbeat as "two clacks of a water-bellows," and later in *De Motu Cordis* (1628), Harvey wrote that " . . . with each motion of the heart when there is the delivery of a quantity of blood from the veins to the arteries . . . a pulse takes place and can be heard within the chest."[14] This description leaves no doubt that Harvey was aware of sounds originating in the beating heart. Robert Hooke was not only familiar with the heart sounds but foresaw the value of clinical auscultation, stating in his Cutlerian Lectures published posthumously in 1705, "I have been able to hear very plainly the beating of a man's heart . . . . Who knows, I say, but that it may be possible to discover the Motions of the Internal Parts of Bodies . . . by the sound they make . . . ."[19] The modern era of cardiac auscultation began in 1816 with René Théophile Hyacinthe Laënnec (Fig. 1–4). Laënnec originally practiced direct auscultation as illustrated in an eighteenth century painting showing Laënnec in the Necker Hospital in Paris sitting at the

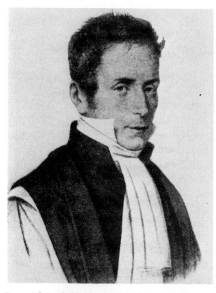

FIGURE 1–4. René Théophile Hyacinthe Laënnec (1781–1826). (Courtesy of Katharine E. Donohue, Special Collections Division, Biomedical Library, UCLA Medical Center.)

bedside with his ear applied to a patient's thorax.[20] Notwithstanding, Laënnec was sensitive to the shortcomings of direct auscultation, writing, "As inconvenient for the physician as for the patient, distaste alone renders it almost impractical in the hospital; it cannot even be proposed to most women and in most of them the volume of the breast is a physical obstacle to its use."[17] The alternative was the stethoscope, the discovery of which is legendary:

In 1816, I was consulted by a young woman labouring under general symptoms of diseased heart, and in whose case percussion and the application of the hand were of little avail on account on her great degree of fatness. The other method just mentioned being rendered inadmissable by age and sex of the patient, I happened to recollect a simple and well-known fact of acoustics, and fancied at the same time, that it might be turned to some use on the present occasion. The fact I allude to is the augmented impression of sound when conveyed through certain solid bodies as when we hear the scratch of the pin at one end of a piece of wood, on applying our ear to the other. Immediately, on this suggestion, I rolled a quire of paper into a sort of cylinder and applied one end of it to the region of the heart and the other to my ear, and was not a little surprised and pleased, to find that I could thereby perceive the action of the heart in a manner much more clear and distinct than I had ever been able to do by the immediate application of the ear. From this moment, I imagined that the circumstance might furnish means for enabling us to ascertain the character, not only of the action of the heart, but of every species of sound produced by the motion of all the thoracic viscera.

The mild ridicule and satiric cartoons that greeted Laënnec's new auscultatory device were soon replaced by an enthusiastic reception, and the London *Times* in September, 1824, announced, "A wonderful instrument called the stethoscope . . . is now in complete vogue in Paris . . . ." Physicians became so attached to the "wonderful instrument" that the soon-to-come flexible binaural stethoscope struggled for recognition. As late as the turn of the century, an article in *Lancet* hotly argued that "the double stethoscope should be altogether done away with . . . ." At the same time, methods for the graphic recording of auscultatory information were moving ahead with the investigations of Otto Frank, Carl Wiggers, and Orias Braun-Menendez. The term "phonocardiogram" came into use, and Einthoven published an account of the string galvanometer for recording heart sounds.[22]

Physical signs elicited from **the thorax** are important adjuncts to the cardiovascular examination and had their origin in Auenbrugger's treatise on percussion.[16]

I here present the Reader with a new sign which I have discovered for detecting diseases of the chest. This consists in Percussion of the human thorax, whereby, according to the character of the particular sounds thence elicited, an opinion is formed of the internal state of that cavity. In making public my discoveries respecting this matter, I have been actuated neither by an itch for writing, nor a fondness for speculation, but by the desire of submitting to my brethren the fruits of seven year's observation and reflection.

Laënnec, in his chapter on pneumothorax in *A Treatise on the Diseases of the Chest*, recalled the dictum of Hippocrates. "Convinced by these symptoms of the existence of a pneumo-thorax combined with a pleuritic effusion, I confidently expected that the Hippocratic succussion of the chest would let us hear the fluctuation of the liquid, and I was not mistaken."[17] Richard C. Cabot's landmark *Physical Diagnosis* (1915) contained three comprehensive chapters on diseases of the lungs and pleural cavity.[23]

In Avicenna's *Canon of Medicine*, dropsy was listed under "cold swellings composed of watery fluid."[24] Whether Avicenna (980–1037) referred to cardiac ascites is open to question, but Withering's account of cure of the dropsy by the Shropshire woman's foxglove leaves little doubt.[25] Nevertheless, well into the twentieth century, Cabot was less than sanguine about **examination of the abdomen**.[23]

> Our methods are crude and inexact compared to those applicable to the chest. Auscultation, despite Canon's brilliant foundation studies, is of practically no use. Inspection is helpful in but few cases. Palpation, our mainstay, is often rendered almost impossible by thickness, muscular spasm, or ticklishness of the abdominal walls. Percussion is of great value in some cases, but yields no useful results in the majority.

REFERENCES

1. Mackenzie, J.: Principles of Diagnosis and Treatment in Heart Affections. London, Oxford University Press, 1916.
2. Linfors, E. W., and Neelson, F. A.: The case for bedside rounds. N. Engl. J. Med. 303:1230, 1980.
3. Cushing, H.: The Life of Sir William Osler. Oxford, The Clarendon Press, 1925.
4. Mackenzie, J.: Diseases of the Heart. London, Henry Frowde, Hodder & Stoughton, 1908.
5. Veith, I.: Huang Ti Nei Ching Su Wen: The Yellow Emperor's Classic of Internal Medicine. Berkeley, University of California Press, 1972.
6. Osler, W.: The Evolution of Modern Medicine. New Haven, Yale University Press, 1921.
7. Reichert, P. P.: The history of the development of cardiology as a medical specialty. Clin. Cardiol. 1:5, 1978.
8. Lancisi, J. M.: Mortu Cordis et Aneurysmabitus. Roma, 1728.
9. Hunter, J.: A Treatise on the Blood, Inflammation, and Gun-Shot Wounds. London, George Nicol, Bookseller to his Majesty, Pall-Mall, 1794.

10. Chauveau, J. B. A., and Marey, E. J.: Appariels et experiences cardiographics. Memoirs Acad. Med. 26:268, 1863.
11. Wiggers, C. J.: The Pressure Pulses in the Cardiovascular System. London, Longmans, Green and Co., 1928.
12. Mackenzie, J.: The Study of the Pulse, Arterial, Venous, and Hepatic, and of the Movements of the Heart. Edinburgh, Young J. Pentland, 1902.
13. Basta, L. L., and Bettinger, J. J.: The cardiac impulse: A new look at an old art. Am. Heart J. 97:96, 1979.
14. Harvey, W.: An Anatomical Disquisition on the Motion of the Heart and Blood in Animals. London, 1628 (translated from the Latin by Robert Willis, Barnes, Surrey, England, 1847). In Willius, F. A., and Keys, T. E.: Classics of Cardiology, Vol. 1, Malabar, Florida, Robert E. Krieger Publishing Co., 1983.
15. Chauveau, J. B. A., and Marey, E. J.: Determination graphiques des rapports de la pulsation cardiaque avec les mouvements de l'oreillette et du ventricle, obtenue au moyen d'un appareil enregistreur. CR Soc Biol (Paris) 13:3, 1861.
16. Auenbrugger, L.: Inventum Novum ex Percussione Thoracis Humani. Vienna, 1761 (translated by John Forbes, London, T. and G. Underwood, Fleet Street, 1824).
17. Laënnec, R. T. H.: A Treatise on the Diseases of the Chest (translated from the French by John Forbes, M.D.). London, T. and G. Underwood, Fleet Street, 1824.
18. McKusick, V. A., Sharp, W. D., and Warner, A. O.: An exhibition on the history of cardiovascular sound including the evolution of the stethoscope. Bull. Hist. Med. 31:463, 1957.
19. Hooke, R.: The Posthumous Works of Robert Hooke, containing his Cutlerian Lectures and Other Discourses Read at the Meeting of the Illustrious Royal Society, etc. In McKusick, V. A.: Cardiovascular Sound. Baltimore, The Williams & Wilkins Co., 1958.
20. Willius, F. A., and Keys, T. E.: Classics of Cardiology, Vol. 1. Malabar, Florida, Robert E. Krieger Publishing Co., 1983, p. 324.
21. Sayers, H. W.: The decay of auscultation and the use of the binaural stethoscope. Lancet 1:369, 1902.
22. Einthoven, W.: Die registrierung des menschlichen herztone mittels des sartengalvanometers. Pflugers Arch. Physiol. 117:461, 1907.
23. Cabot, R. C.: Physical Diagnosis. 6th Ed. New York, William Wood and Company, 1915.
24. Gruner, O. C.: A Treatise on the Canon of Avicenna. London, Luzac & Co., 1930.
25. Withering, W.: An Account of the Foxglove and Some of its Medical Uses. Birmingham, M. Swinney, 1785.

PHYSICAL APPEARANCE

The eye . . . is the chief means whereby the understanding may most fully and abundantly appreciate the infinite works of nature.

LEONARDO DA VINCI

Inspection deals with what the eye sees—the patient's physical appearance, general and detailed. In order "to see," however, the physician's eye must be trained. "The 'innocent eye' which should see the world afresh (does) not see it at all."[1]

Many distinctive physical appearances predict specific coexisting cardiac diseases, whereas other appearances are *caused* by cardiac or vascular disorders. The examiner should first pay attention to *general* appearance, then to *details* (Table 2–1). I shall select for emphasis examples of practical interest; no attempt will be made to be comprehensive. My purpose, instead, is to instill the discipline of systematic assessment of physical appearance as an integral part of the clinical examination of the heart and circulation. In so doing, I shall deal in turn with (1) general somatic features, (2) gestures and gait, and (3) detailed appearance of face, eyes, mouth, hands, feet, skin, muscles, tendons, thorax, and abdomen.

GENERAL APPEARANCE

General appearance often distinguishes at a glance acute from chronic illness. Conversely, the patient may

13

TABLE 2–1. Physical Appearance

General appearance
Gestures and gait
Detailed appearance
    Face
    Eyes—external and internal
    Mouth—external and internal
    Hands and feet
    Skin
    Muscles and tendons
    Thorax
    Abdomen

look well despite the presence or presumed presence of cardiac or vascular disease. The picture of certain **acute illnesses** is familiar. Pulmonary edema is dramatically recognized in the struggling, frightened, diaphoretic patient, dyspneic while sitting bolt upright. Or witness the patient with an acute myocardial infarction—anxious, ashen, diaphoretic, reacting to oppressive chest pain with all of its real and symbolic meanings. The picture of cardiogenic shock, familiar to us all, was described by Shakespeare in the death of Falstaff.[2]

> So he cried out, 'God, God!' three or four times. Now I, to comfort him, bid him he should not think of God; I hoped that there is no need to trouble himself with any such thoughts yet. So he bade me lay more clothes on his feet; I put my hand into the bed and felt them and they were as cold as any stone; I then felt to his knees; and they were as cold as any stone and so upward and upward, all was as cold as any stone.

The general appearance of **chronic illness** is exemplified by the catabolic effects of protracted congestive heart failure—wasted pectoral, shoulder girdle, and arm muscles, edematous legs, protruding ascitic abdomen, drawn face. The appearance of the "coronary-prone" patient is a stereotype—the mesomorphic, balding, hirsute, middle-aged, overweight male of good appetite whose fingers are stained with nicotine, whose ashtray is filled with the butts of cigarettes that preceded the one he is smoking, while close at hand is a briefcase bulging with papers, symbols of deadlines he feels driven to meet.

The general appearance of thyrotoxicosis can be distinctive—a lean, tremulous individual with quick movements and "bright eyes" with or without exophthalmos, but with rapid atrial fibrillation or sinus tachycardia (see later). The patient with *hypo*thyroidism (see below) is the antithesis—lethargic and pallid, with slow movements, coarse features, and bradycardia.

Patients may be distinctively tall (gigantism) or distinctively short (dwarfism). The general appearance of the Marfan syndrome is an example of the former[3]—a strikingly tall patient with excessively long extremities (see below) and sparse subcutaneous fat—predicting the presence of aortic root disease and myxomatous degeneration of the mitral valve and annulus. Gigantism in the neonate is represented by the infant of the diabetic mother (Fig. 2–1). The description of James W. Farquhar suffices:[4]

> The infants are remarkable not only because, like foetal versions of Shadrach, Meshach and Abednego, they emerge at least alive from within the fiery metabolic furnace of diabetes mellitus, but because they resemble one another so closely that they might well be related. They are plump, sleek, liberally coated with vernix caseosa, full-faced and plethoric. The umbilical cord and the placenta share in the gigantism. During their first 24 or more extra-uterine hours they lie on their backs, bloated and flushed, their legs flexed and abducted, their lightly closed hands on each side of the head, the abdomen prominent and their respiration sighing. They convey a distinct impression of having had such a surfeit of both food and fluid pressed upon them by an insistent hostess that they desire only peace so that they may recover from their excesses.

Short stature is seen in the 45 XO Turner syndrome (Fig. 2–2A) represented by a phenotypic female with webbing of the neck, sexual infantilism (absent or scanty pubic and axillary hair), wide-set nipples, low hairline, small chin, and wide carrying angles of the arms.[5] The "female Turner" (45 XO) predicts the presence of coarctation of the aorta and bicuspid aortic valve. Another Turner phenotype is seen in the Noonan syndrome with normal chromosomal composition (46 XX female, 46 XY male) (Fig. 2–2B), but the cardiac disease is likely to be pulmonic valve stenosis, often a dysplastic valve.[5]

The appearance of obesity varies and should be carefully characterized. The combination of somnolence and obesity, known as the pickwickian syndrome, was so

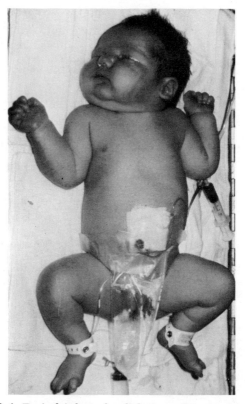

FIGURE 2–1. Typical infant of a diabetic mother showing neonatal "gigantism": plump, full-faced, plethoric, bloated, and flushed.

named by C. Sidney Burwell[6] based upon the description of Charles Dickens' fat boy (Fig. 2–3A).

A most violent and startling knocking was heard at the door . . . . The object that presented itself to the eyes of the astonished clerk was a boy—a wonderfully fat boy—standing upright on the mat, with his eyes closed as if in sleep. He had never seen such a fat boy . . . , and this, coupled with the utter calmness and repose of his appearance, so very different from what was reasonably to have been expected of the inflictor of such knocks, smote him with wonder . . . . The extraordinary boy spoke not a word; but he nodded once and seemed to the clerk's imagination to snore feebly.

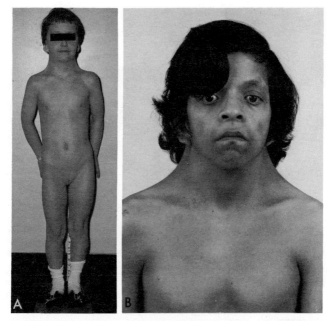

FIGURE 2–2. *A*, A 13-year-old girl with 45 XO Turner syndrome and coarctation of the aorta. She exhibits short stature, webbing of the neck, absence of pubic hair, wide-set nipples, and small chin. *B*, An 18-year-old boy with 46 XY Noonan syndrome with pulmonic stenosis and an atrial septal defect. He shows typical webbing of the neck.

Alveolar hypoventilation that accompanies pickwickian obesity results in hypercapnea, somnolence (Fig. 2–3B), hypoxemia, increased pulmonary vascular resistance, and pulmonary hypertension. By contrast, the obesity of Cushing's syndrome predicts the presence of **systemic hypertension,** not pulmonary hypertension. The Cushingoid appearance is typified by central obesity with rounding of the face, thick fat pads in the supraclavicular fossae, and a marked increase in thoracoabdominal panniculus. Abdominal obesity can advance to grotesque proportions while the extremities remain remarkably slender.

Gestures and gait are sometimes important features of physical appearance. A clenched fist pressed against the

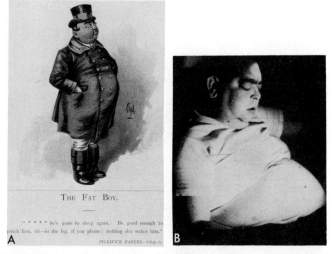

FIGURE 2–3. *A*, Charles Dickens' *Fat Boy*. (Courtesy of Professor Ada Nisbet, Department of English, University of California, Los Angeles.) *B*, An obese 32-year-old man with the pickwickian syndrome photographed by the author as the patient fell asleep while his history was being taken.

sternum is a time-honored gesture employed to describe the oppressive pain of myocardial infarction. The importance of observing gait was emphasized by James Mackenzie:[7] "When the patient presents . . . for examination, the physician naturally scrutinizes him and makes a mental note of his gait . . . and how he deports himself generally." Contemporary physicians, except for neurologists, seldom routinely watch their patients walk, even though an abnormal gait may be the first evidence of a systemic neuromuscular disease with cardiac involvement. Pseudohypertrophic Duchenne muscular dystrophy, for example, results in a characteristic slow, clumsy, waddling gait caricatured by exaggerated lumbar lordosis and protuberant abdomen (Fig. 2–4). When the child is asked to rise from a recumbent position, he is apt to use the distinctive gestures originally described by Gowers[5]

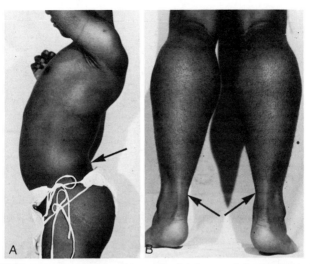

FIGURE 2–4. *A*, A young boy with classic pseudohypertrophic X-linked Duchenne muscular dystrophy and the typical exaggerated lumbar lordosis *(arrow)*. *B*, There is striking calf pseudohypertrophy with shortening of the Achilles tendons *(arrows)*, causing the patient to stand on his toes. The boy had regional dystrophy of the posterobasal left ventricular wall.

(Fig. 2–5). The cardiac involvement in Duchenne dystrophy targets the posterobasal left ventricular wall.

DETAILED APPEARANCE

"For by his face straight shall you know his heart."[8]

Facial Expression. Facial expressions may convey anxiety or calm. Apprehension provokes a variety of cardiocirculatory disturbances in persons without organic heart disease, or anxiety may result from fear of real or imagined cardiac disease. The face is often a barometer of age, appearing chronologically appropriate or inappropriate. Premature aging takes one of its most dramatic forms in Werner's syndrome[9] (Fig. 2–6A), a disorder characterized in part by premature graying of the hair,

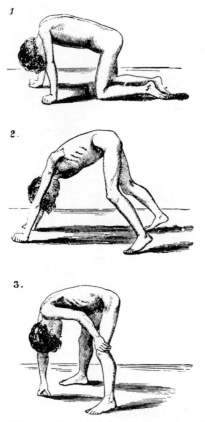

FIGURE 2–5. Gowers' sign. "Mode of rising from the ground in pseudohypertrophic paralysis," as originally described and published in Gowers, WR: Diseases of the Nervous System. Philadelphia, P. Blakiston, Son & Co, 1888, p 383.

frontal baldness in males, taut skin, beaking of the nose, and cataracts. Coronary artery disease and systemic atherosclerosis are strikingly premature. A dramatic variation on this theme occurs in children with the alopecia and senile appearance of the Hutchinson-Gilford syndrome of premature aging (Fig. 2–6*B*), in which childhood atherosclerosis and death from cardiac infarction are not uncommon. Patients with myotonic muscular dystrophy

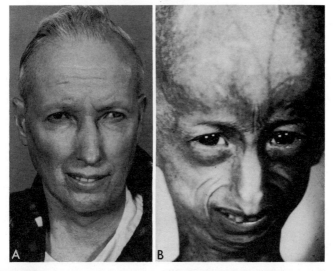

FIGURE 2–6. *A*, A 34-year-old man with the typical premature aging of Werner's syndrome. There is graying of the hair, frontal baldness, and a cataract in the left eye. Atrophic skin is pulled tightly over the bridge of the nose. *B*, A 10-year-old boy with the Hutchinson-Gilford syndrome—progeria (premature aging) with nanism (dwarfism). There is complete alopecia and tight, atrophic skin. The child died of a myocardial infarction.

appear prematurely old, with graying of the hair, frontal thinning or baldness even in females, early cataracts, and an expressionless, myopathic facies (Fig. 2–7). Abnormalities of cardiac impulse formation and conduction are features.

A facial "butterfly rash" with malar depigmentation point to the diagnosis of systemic lupus erythematosus with involvement of endocardium, myocardium, and pericardium. In the carcinoid syndrome, a cardinal facial appearance is the dramatic flushing. The sudden bright red to violaceous hue may be accompanied by facial and periorbital edema; during the flush, severe hypotension, even shock, sometimes occurs. Cardiac involvement usually takes the form of pulmonic stenosis and tricuspid stenosis/regurgitation.

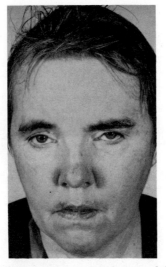

FIGURE 2–7. Expressionless, myopathic facies and thin frontal hair in a woman with myotonic muscular dystrophy. Cataracts were present but are not seen in this photograph.

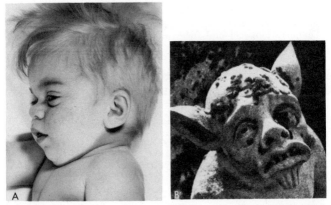

FIGURE 2–8. *A,* Typical coarse physiognomy of a child with the Hurler syndrome (gargoylism). At necropsy, the mitral leaflets were thickened and there was severe narrowing of the lumens of the coronary arteries. (Courtesy of Dr. Hans Zellweger, University of Iowa, Iowa City.) *B,* Gargoyle showing the grotesque features, especially bulging eyes, prominent supraorbital ridges, blunt upturned nose, thick lips, and peg teeth. (Courtesy of Professor Robbert Flick, Department of Fine Arts, University of Southern California, Los Angeles.)

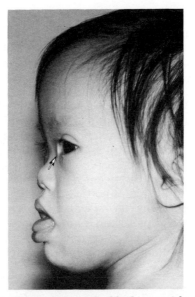

FIGURE 2–9. Profile of a 17-month-old Chinese girl with Down syndrome. Arrow identifies the typical inner epicanthic fold in addition to the normal horizontal Asian fold above the outer canthus. The nose is flat with depressed nasal bridge, and the tongue is typically protuberant.

Facial appearance in hypothyroidism is characterized by dull, coarse features, an enlarged tongue, thickened skin, dry hair that does not curl, puffy eyelids, and sparse eyebrows, the outer thirds of which may be absent. Pericardial effusion is common, and the accompanying hyperlipidemia is held responsible for premature coronary artery disease.

In the Hurler syndrome, the term "gargoylism" refers to the grotesque facial features that are recognizable at a glance (Fig. 2–8A). The skull is malformed, the supraorbital ridges are prominent, the bridge of the nose is depressed, the lips are thick, and the teeth are peg-shaped as in a gargoyle (Fig. 2–8B). The Hurler syndrome is a variety of mucopolysaccharidosis that involves the mitral and aortic valves (regurgitation and/or stenosis) together with thickening of the walls and narrowing of the lumina of the coronary arteries.[10]

A number of facial appearances predict specific or relatively specific **congenital cardiac or vascular anomalies.** Figure 2–9 shows the face of a 17-month-old Chinese girl with Down syndrome (trisomy 21). The profile exhibits the typical flat nose and nasal bridge, the large protuberant tongue, and the inner epicanthic skin fold in addition to the normal horizontal Asian epicanthic fold above the outer canthus. Down syndrome is usually accompanied by an endocardial cushion defect.[5] Another distinctive facial appearance is a feature of children with nonfamilial supravalvular aortic stenosis and pulmonary arterial stenosis. The face is characterized by a large mouth, patulous lips, small chin, baggy cheeks, blunt upturned nose, wide-set eyes, and malformed teeth (Fig. 2–10). The fetal alcohol syndrome (in offspring of heavy

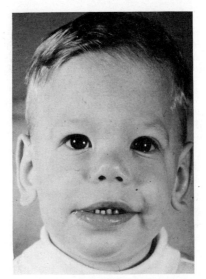

FIGURE 2–10. Facial appearance of a boy with bilateral stenosis of the pulmonary arteries, supravalvular aortic stenosis, mental retardation, and infantile hypercalcemia. The chin is small, the mouth large, the lips patulous, the nose blunt and upturned, the eyes wideset, the forehead broad, the cheeks baggy, and the teeth malformed.

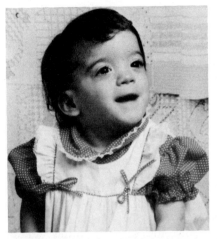

FIGURE 2–11. Fetal alcohol syndrome physiognomy in a 21-month-old girl with a ventricular septal defect and pulmonic stenosis. She exhibits micrognathia, absent philtrum, short palpebral fissures, and epicanthal folds. (Courtesy of Dr. David A. Ferry, Encino, California.)

maternal drinkers) results in short palpebral fissures, a hypoplastic upper lip with thin vermilion, diminished to absent philtrum, micrognathia, and midfacial growth deficiency[11] (Fig. 2–11). Coexisting congenital cardiac malformations usually take the form of atrial septal defect or ventricular septal defect alone or with pulmonic stenosis. The cardiofacial syndrome consists of distinctive unilateral partial lower facial weakness that appears only when the patient cries.[12] The associated type of cardiac anomaly varies, but ventricular septal defect is the most common.

External and Internal Appearance of the Eyes. Examination of the eyes externally is an extension of the examination of the face. External features of the eyes can usually be assessed with the unaided senses and a pocket flashlight. While some abnormalities are recognizable at a glance (strabismus or conspicuous exophthalmos), detection of other abnormalities requires careful inspection of lids, lacrimal glands, palpebral fissures, eyebrows, conjunctivae, sclerae, cornea, iris, and lens.

The **bulbus oculi** (ocular bulb or eyeball) is normally contained well within its bony cavity, the orbit. In hyperthyroidism, the appearance of the ocular bulb varies from symmetric or asymmetric protrusion (exophthalmos) to mild lid retraction and stare. These appearances shed light on otherwise unexplained rapid atrial fibrillation, angina pectoris, or high-output heart failure. In euthyroid patients, slight proptosis and stare are occasionally due to chronic elevation of systemic venous pressure; when severe tricuspid regurgitation coexists, the proptosis may be accompanied by systolic anterior movement of the eyeballs, best detected when the examiner observes the eyes with an oblique light while the patient looks forward from a sitting position. Conversely, *shrunken* eyeballs result when the catabolic effects of chronic congestive heart failure cause loss of retro-orbital fat and connective tissue in adults. Nystagmus—involuntary lateral gaze oscillations of the eyeball—is a feature of Friedreich's ataxia, which may be accompanied by hypertrophic or dilated cardiomyopathy.

The **eyelids** themselves sometimes disclose telltale signs. A common example is represented by xanthalasma, which are circumscribed, yellowish plaques that contain cholesterol. Xanthalasma are detected near the inner canthus and are best seen when the eyelids are gently closed. Their presence, especially in young adults, arouses suspicion of atherosclerotic coronary artery disease. Lid-lag, another ocular feature of hyperthyroidism (see above), is characterized by visible sclera superior to the iris as movement of the upper lid lags behind the eyeball on downward gaze. Ptosis, often asymmetric, is part of the external ophthalmoplegia and pigmentary retinopathy of the Kearns-Sayre syndrome (Fig. 2–12), which is associated with abnormalities of infranodal conduction culminating in complete heart block.[13] In sarcoidosis, enlarged lacrimal glands sometimes obviously protrude behind the lateral margins of the upper lids (Fig. 2–13). Eversion of the upper lid permits direct inspection of the enlarged lacrimal glands. Sarcoid involves the heart either secondarily by causing pulmonary hypertension or primarily by infiltrating the conduction

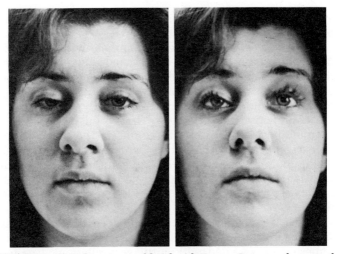

FIGURE 2–12. Eighteen-year-old girl with Kearns-Sayre syndrome and bilateral asymmetric ptosis. She also had pigmentary retinopathy and bifascicular block.

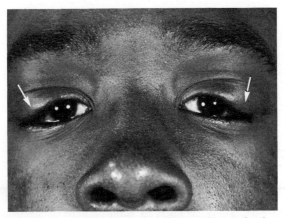

FIGURE 2–13. A young boy with sarcoidosis and typical enlargement of the lacrimal glands causing protrusion of the lateral aspects of the upper lids *(arrows)*.

system (especially the atrioventricular junction and His bundle) and the myocardium.[14]

The **conjunctivae** are best examined with a pocket flashlight as the lower lid is retracted downward while the patient looks up. The pallor of anemia or the suffusion of cyanosis becomes apparent. White-centered petechiae of infective endocarditis are most readily identified on the conjunctiva of the everted lower lid (Fig. 2–14A). Conjunctivitis with urethritis points to the diagnosis of Reiter's disease, with involvement in the acute stage taking the form of pericarditis and abnormalities in atrioventricular (AV) conduction, while the chronic manifestations are represented by AV block and aortic regurgitation.

The **sclera** can disclose a finding as pedestrian as jaundice or as unusual as the blue sclerae of osteogenesis imperfecta associated with aortic regurgitation[16] (see below). Examination of the **cornea** may disclose corneal arcus which, when present in relatively young patients (Fig. 2–15), prompts suspicion of coronary artery disease.

The appearance of the **iris** in Down syndrome may reveal distinctive Brushfield spots, a circle of punctate, depigmented dots circumferentially arranged at the pe-

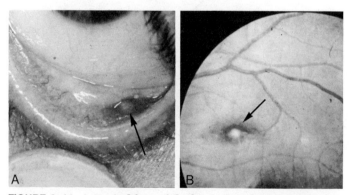

FIGURE 2–14. *A,* Typical lower lid white-centered conjunctival petechia (arrow) in a young man with infective endocarditis of the aortic valve. *B,* Retinal Roth spot (white center) *(arrow)* surrounded by hemorrhage in a young woman with mitral valve infective endocarditis.

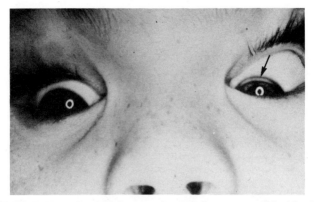

FIGURE 2–15. Left corneal arcus *(arrow)* in a 4-year-old girl with homozygous familial hypercholesterolemia.

riphery of the iris[5] (Fig. 2–16*A*). Brushfield spots are not seen in patients with darkly pigmented irises. Congenital coloboma or fissures of the iris result in a change in pupillary shape from circular to oblong, creating the appearance of a "cat eye"[17] (Fig. 2–17). The most common coexisting congenital cardiac malformations in the "cat

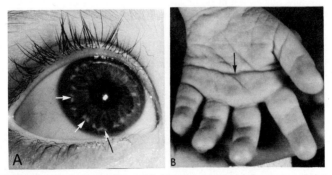

FIGURE 2–16. *A,* Typical Brushfield spots (circle of depigmented dots along the outer circumference of the iris, *arrows*) and sparse, thin eyelashes in a child with Down syndrome and a partial endocardial cushion defect. *B,* The hand of a 6-month-old child with Down syndrome and complete endocardial cushion defect. A simian crease *(arrow)* traverses the palm.

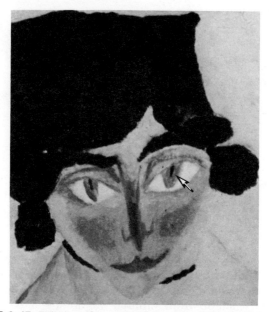

FIGURE 2–17. Painting of a woman's head by Lyonel Feininger, an American-born German Expressionist artist. I believe that the model had congenital coloboma (fissures) of the iris *(arrow)* causing the "cat's eye" appearance. In the original painting, the cheeks have a reddish blue hue, suggesting cyanotic congenital heart disease, probably Fallot's tetralogy based upon the estimated age of the subject.

eye syndrome" include Fallot's tetralogy, tricuspid atresia, and isolated defects in the atrial or ventricular septum.[5]

The appearance of the **pupils**—size, shape, reaction to light, and accommodation—is diagnostically important. In diabetes mellitus, the pupils are sometimes unequal and nonreactive to light. The distinctive Argyll Robertson pupil, which is small, irregular, and usually bilateral, constricts to convergence accommodation but not to light and is a feature of neurosyphilis (tabes dorsalis), often accompanied by aortic regurgitation.[18]

A common abnormal appearance of the **lens** is the cataract. Premature cataracts occur in myotonic muscular dystrophy (Fig. 2–7), in Werner's syndrome (Fig. 2–6A), and in offspring of mothers with first trimester rubella.[5] Subluxation of the lens is an important feature of the Marfan syndrome (Fig. 2–18) and homocystinuria.[3] The unsupported lens imparts a distinctive shimmer to a transverse light beam when lateral motion of the eye is abruptly halted, an observation best made with the patient sitting in a relatively dark room. In the Marfan syndrome, the lens dislocation is typically **upward** (Fig. 2–18), whereas in homocystinuria, downward dislocation is the rule.[3] Cardiac involvement in the Marfan syndrome was commented upon earlier. Homocystinuria is accompanied by arterial and venous thromboses, myocardial infarction, and pulmonary embolism.

Examination of the **internal appearance** of the eye—retina, retinal arteries, retinal veins, and optic disc—requires an ophthalmoscope. Skilled use of this instrument is therefore a necessary part of the cardiac and vascular physical examination. The optic fundi provide visual access to the small arteries, arterioles, veins, venules, and capillaries. The appearance of hypertensive retinopathy is well known. The permanent or relatively permanent changes consist of increased light reflex, copper wire appearance, arteriovenous nicking, increased

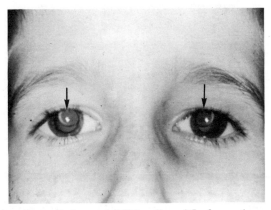

FIGURE 2–18. Typical *upward* dislocation of the lenses *(arrows)* in a young woman with the Marfan syndrome.

tortuosity, and irregular caliber of the arterioles. Other changes tend to disappear with control of blood pressure and are represented by hemorrhages, exudates, cotton-wool patches, and papilledema. Less well known in hypertensive patients is the distinctive appearance of retinal arteries when the hypertension is due to coarctation of the aorta.[5] The retinal arteries show frequent "U turns" (Fig. 2–19) but virtually never the changes of hypertensive retinopathy.[5]

Retinal arterial emboli sometimes have characteristic appearances that reveal their sources. Calcific emboli tend to be white, dull, and in close proximity to the disc margin. Cholesterol emboli (Hollenhorst plaques) are highly refractile. Fibrin-platelet emboli appear as whitish plugs that are sometimes seen moving through the retinal arteries.

In cyanotic congenital heart disease, *retinal veins* are often large in caliber, even toward the periphery, because of the increase in red cell mass. Occasionally, papilledema and retinal edema occur in these patients in response to the low systemic arterial oxygen saturation.

Retinal Roth spots in infective endocarditis have a white, "cotton-wool" appearance (perivascular collec-

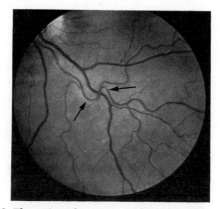

FIGURE 2–19. The retina of a 28-year-old woman with coarctation of the aorta. Arrows point to typical U-shaped tortuosity of a retinal artery. There are no changes of hypertensive retinopathy.

tions of lymphocytes in the nerve layer of the retina) surrounded by hemorrhage (see Fig. 2–14B). Bilateral atypical pigmentary retinopathy is a feature of the Kearns-Sayre syndrome mentioned above.[13] The dramatic appearance of retinal detachment is an occasional feature of the Ehlers-Danlos syndrome that is associated with mitral and aortic regurgitation and dissecting aneurysm.[3] Angioid streaks are another retinal feature of the Ehlers-Danlos syndrome and radiate from the optic discs as reddish brown or gray lines conspicuously wider than the retinal vessels.[3] Angioid streaks also occur in pseudoxanthoma elasticum (with renal artery involvement, systemic hypertension, premature calcification of systemic and coronary arteries), Paget's bone disease (high output congestive heart failure), and sickle cell anemia (pulmonary hypertension and occlusion of small intramyocardial arteries).

External and Internal Appearance of the Mouth. Examination of the mouth includes the lips, mucous membranes, teeth, gums, tongue, and palate. The color of the lips may disclose the pallor of anemia or the bluish color of cyanosis. Thick lips are features of the Hurler syndrome (see Fig. 2–8) mentioned earlier. Attention has already been called to the absent philtrum of the fetal alcohol syndrome (see Fig. 2–11).

Mucous membrane lesions are observed by everting the upper or lower lip and by inspecting the mucosa of the oral cavity with a flashlight. Petechiae of infective endocarditis can be identified. In hereditary telangiectasia (Rendu-Osler-Weber syndrome), clusters of small ruby patches appear on the lips, mucous membranes, palate, and tongue (Fig. 2–20) and are associated with pulmonary arteriovenous fistulae.[5] The appearance of these mucuous membrane lesions was vividly described in an annotation from *Lancet*:[19]

Every large general hospital is certain to have on its list of frequent attenders a small group of unfortunate adults who come to the casualty department complaining of recurrent bleeding from the nose, lips or mouth. The blood is seen to stem from an insignificant leak in the center of a small ruby patch, many of which are usually to be found gathered here and there on mucous membranes (Fig.

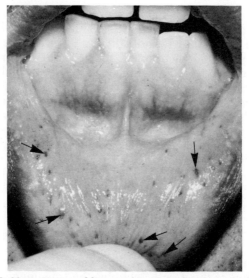

FIGURE 2–20. A 28-year-old man whose lower lip is everted to show clusters of the typical discrete ruby patches *(arrows)* of Rendu-Osler-Weber hereditary hemorrhagic telangiectasia. Bilateral pulmonary arteriovenous fistulas were present.

2–20). Although the flow of blood is seldom vigorous, it may eventually by its persistence, draw some concern. Its arrest can be infuriatingly difficult. Each ruby patch marks the position of a tiny arteriovenous communication at the capillary level. Whatever the cause, they can be induced to bleed by the most trivial of injuries.

An important aspect of the examination of the mouth is the **oral hygiene** of teeth and gums in patients with cardiac or vascular lesions susceptible to infective endocarditis. **Malformations** of the teeth are diagnostically important in the nonhereditary form of supravalvular aortic stenosis with pulmonary artery stenosis (see Fig. 2–10). Abnormal, peg teeth are common in the Hurler syndrome (gargoylism) (see Fig. 2–8). An even more distinctive malformation of the teeth is a feature of the Ellis–van Creveld syndrome in which abnormal, prematurely erupted teeth are often present at birth, in addition to gingival hypertrophy and multiple frenula.[5] When phenytoin is used as an antiarrhythmic, a side effect is gingival hyperplasia.

The appearance of the **tongue** should be judged according to size, texture, position, and specific surface lesions. A large, protruding tongue is common in Down syndrome (see Fig. 2–9) and in Hurler syndrome mentioned above. An odd variation on the theme is the glossoptosis (retraction of the tongue) that occurs with the Pierre Robin syndrome and may cause upper airway obstruction and pulmonary hypertension.[20]

Examination of the **hard palate** may disclose the innocuous torus palatinus (a bony protuberance or ridge sometimes found at the junction of the intermaxillary and transverse palatine sutures). A distinctive and often dramatically high-arched palate is a feature of the Marfan syndrome.[3]

The Hands and the Feet. After the face, the hands are the most expressive parts of the human body. A thumb capable of apposing each finger was a major step forward in mammalian evolution. Strictly speaking, the hand is equipped with four fingers (triphalangeal digits) and one thumb (a biphalangeal digit). For the purpose of the following discussion, the hands and feet will be considered together. Their appearances are assessed in terms of color and texture of the skin, structure, and the presence of discrete lesions.

An abnormality of color is represented by **cyanosis** (Gr. *kyanos* = blue, *osis* = condition). In infants, children, and young adults, cyanosis accompanied by clubbing (Fig. 2–21) is typically in response to right-to-left shunts of cyanotic congenital heart disease. In older adults, these signs may accompany the cyanotic cor pulmonale of advanced chronic obstructive lung disease.

Cyanosis and clubbing are diagnostically important not only because of their presence and degree, but also because of their *distribution*. Cyanosis and clubbing equally distributed in the hands and feet indicate that the right-to-left shunt is proximal to the brachiocephalic arteries as they leave the aortic root. Conversely, specific diagnostic connotations are associated with *differential* cyanosis and clubbing, a term that by convention refers

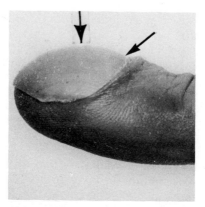

FIGURE 2–21. Typical profile of a finger with marked clubbing and cyanosis. The dorsum of the nail is not only abnormally convex *(vertical arrow)*, but the angle at its base is absent *(oblique arrow)*.

to cyanosis and clubbing that are present in the feet but not in the hands. The diagnostic implication of differential cyanosis is a right-to-left shunt that delivers unoxygenated blood from the pulmonary trunk into the aorta *distal* to the left subclavian artery, so the toes are cyanosed and clubbed but the hands are spared (Fig. 2–22). Patent ductus arteriosus with suprasystemic pulmonary vascular resistance is the cause.[5] Differential cyanosis and clubbing are best observed when the patient sits with knees flexed and hands placed upon the dorsa of the feet, as shown in Figure 2–22. Differential cyanosis is heightened by exercise or by immersion of the hands and feet in warm water. Exercise increases the right-to-left shunt, and warmth increases skin blood flow.

Normal individuals, generally young women, sometimes have *peripheral* cyanosis, especially of the feet, because of simple vasoconstriction. The feet are conspicuously cooler than the hands. Diagnostic error can be prevented by warming the hands and feet, an intervention that abolishes peripheral cyanosis but exaggerates central cyanosis, as noted in the preceding paragraph.

True **digital clubbing** in cyanotic patients (see Fig. 2–21) differs from an increase in the convexity of an oth-

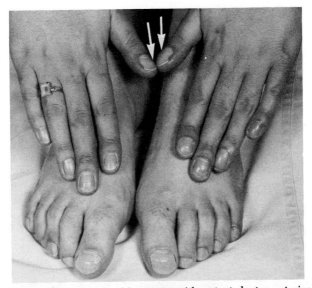

FIGURE 2–22. A 28-year-old woman with patent ductus arteriosus, pulmonary hypertension, and reversed shunt. She is sitting with her hands placed on the dorsa of her feet in order to compare the fingers and toes. The right hand is acyanotic and the fingers are not clubbed. The left hand exhibits mild cyanosis with clubbing (compare the two thumbs, *arrows*). The toes are frankly cyanosed and clubbed.

erwise normal nail.[21] Clubbing requires sufficient elevation of the base of the nail to eliminate the angle between the base and contiguous soft tissue, as shown in Figure 2–21. Clubbing therefore consists not only of an exaggeration of the normal convexity of the nail but of an extension of that convexity to the *base* of the nail. Clubbing is best detected, especially when subtle, by observing the digit in profile (see Fig. 2–21). In addition, the nail's elevated base has a spongy texture that is detected by applying light pressure.

A minor variation on the theme of cyanosis takes the form of "tuft" erythema of the fingertips that sometimes precedes cyanosis in patients with small or intermittent right-to-left shunts.[5] In a very different setting, a bright red painless flush of the palms and fingers sometimes

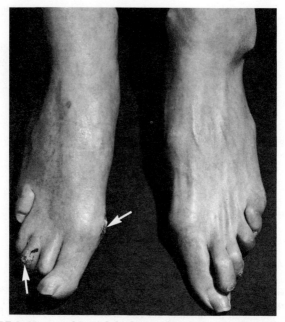

FIGURE 2–23. Atrophic, tightly drawn skin, ischemic ulcers *(arrows)*, and hypoplastic nails in a patient with severe peripheral vascular disease associated with the premature aging of Werner's syndrome (see Fig. 2–6*A*).

occurs months after an acute cardiac infarction. The mechanism is unclear, although the temporal relation to the infarct is well established. The fingertips are typically bright red but are painless and without clubbing.

In the presence of the protein-losing enteropathy of chronic constrictive pericarditis, hypoalbuminemic "stripes"—alternating dark and light lines parallel to the tips of the nails—are sometimes seen.[21] A much more common cause of these nail stripes is Laënnec's cirrhosis.

Changes in **texture** as well as color of the skin of the feet and toes are features of peripheral vascular disease (see Chapter 3). The atrophic skin is shiny and tightly drawn (Fig. 2–23). An ischemic foot is typically pallid

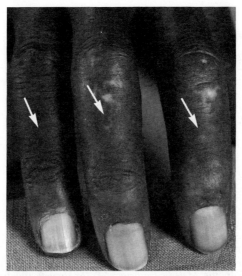

FIGURE 2–24. Hands of a 56-year-old woman with progressive systemic sclerosis and pulmonary hypertension. The photograph shows characteristic smooth, thickened skin of the fingers *(arrows)* with loss of the fine transverse creases.

when the leg is elevated and bright red (rubor) when the leg is dependent.

Raynaud's phenomenon, sometimes seen in primary pulmonary hypertension, is characterized by intermittent alterations in color of the fingers, less commonly of toes. The affected digits initially manifest intense pallor followed by frank cyanosis; before restitution of normal color, the digits may develop intense rubor (reactive hyperemia).

In the post–myocardial infarction shoulder-hand syndrome, the skin over the dorsa of the hands and fingers becomes swollen, tense and discolored, with subsequent wrinkling and Dupuytren's contractures.[22] In progressive systemic sclerosis (scleroderma) a change in texture of the dorsa of the fingers takes the form of thickened skin with loss of the fine transverse creases (Fig. 2–24). Interstitial pulmonary fibrosis is associated with pulmonary hypertension in progressive systemic sclerosis.

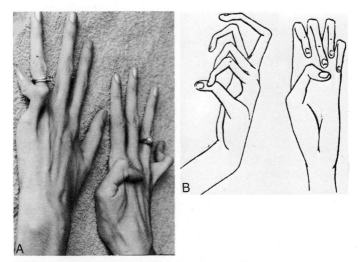

FIGURE 2–25. *A*, The elongated, hyperextensible fingers of a young woman with the Marfan syndrome. *B*, Analogous illustration from Marfan's original paper (Bull Mém Soc Méd Hôp Paris 13:220, 1896).

Abnormalities of structure of the hands and feet may be sufficiently distinctive to establish a high-probability somatic diagnosis and by inference to predict the coexisting cardiac disease. A prime example is the Marfan syndrome with the remarkable appearance of the hands—arachnodactyly and hyperextensible joints (Fig. 2–25).[3] In osteogenesis imperfecta, another heritable disorder of connective tissue[16] (see above), the joints of the hands are hyperextensible, but the fingers are not elongated (Fig. 2–26). Jaccoud's arthritis (sometimes mistaken for rheumatoid arthritis) is a post–rheumatic fever abnormality in which the "deformity" can be voluntarily corrected because the cause is subluxation of the joints rather than erosion and fusion of their articular surfaces[23] (Fig. 2–27).

The hands in Down syndrome are characterized by a simian palmar crease, distal position of the triaxial radius, increased space between the fourth and fifth fingers, and a short fifth finger that is curved inward[5] (see Fig. 2–16B). The association of Down syndrome with endocar-

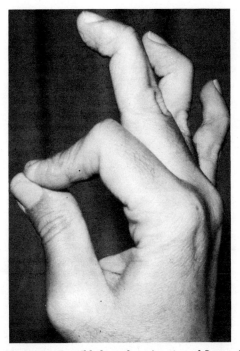

FIGURE 2–26. Hyperextensible but otherwise normal fingers in a young man with osteogenesis imperfecta and aortic regurgitation.

dial cushion defect was mentioned earlier. In the Hurler syndrome (see Fig. 2–8), inward curvature of the fourth and fifth fingers results in a clawlike appearance of the hands, which are wider than they are long.[10] Broad thumbs and toes are characteristic of the Rubinstein-Taybi syndrome,[24] in which the most common coexisting cardiac malformation is patent ductus arteriosus.

Abnormalities of structure of the hands and feet sometimes take the form of accessory digits or deficient digits. The extra digit of polydactyly is almost always an accessory finger, as in the Ellis–van Creveld syndrome, which is accompanied by total anomalous pulmonary venous connection as mentioned above.[5] The fingernails are dysplastic, and the fourth toe frequently overlaps the fifth.

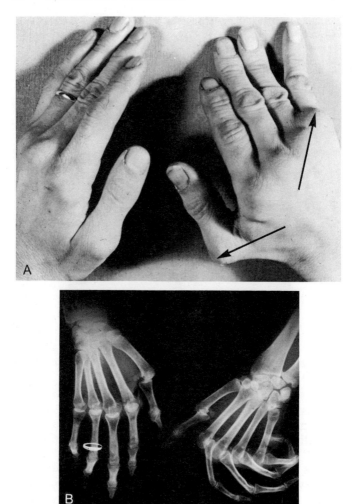

FIGURE 2–27. *A*, Hands of a young man with post–rheumatic fever (Jaccoud's) arthritis. The right hand shows flexion subluxation and ulnar deviation at the metacarpophalangeal joints *(arrows)*; in the left hand, the deformity has been voluntarily corrected. *B*, Comparable radiograph.

The converse of polydactyly is a *decrease* in the number of digits, generally the thumb, as in the Holt-Oram syndrome.[25] The thumb may be present but hypoplastic with an accessory phalanx (triphalangism) that gives the digit a crooked appearance and makes apposition with the fingertips difficult. The Holt-Oram hand defect becomes more obvious when the patient turns the palms up (supination). The most common coexisting cardiac anomaly is an ostium secundum atrial septal defect.[5]

Pes cavus with hammer toe (Fig. 2–28) is a structural abnormality of the foot in Friedreich's ataxia[26] (see above). An even more distinctive and diagnostically useful structural abnormality of the foot is the "rocker-bottom" appearance caused by the protruding heel in trisomy 18, which is usually associated with patent ductus arteriosus or ventricular septal defect.[5]

Discrete lesions of the hands and feet may be subtle and relatively unimportant, such as subungual splinter hemorrhages, the diagnostic specificity of which is low. Conversely, white-centered petechiae of infective endocarditis are significant diagnostic signs (Fig. 2–29). In such patients, Osler's nodes and Janeway lesions should be sought. Osler's nodes are tender, pea-sized, raised, swollen areas most often on the pads of the fingers or

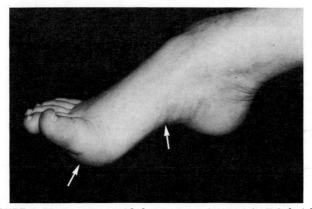

FIGURE 2–28. Pes cavus with hammer toe *(arrows)* in Friedreich's ataxia.

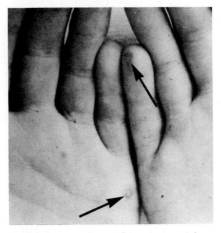

FIGURE 2–29. White-centered petechiae *(arrows)* in a patient with infective endocarditis.

toes, on the thenar or hypothenar eminences, or on the soles of the feet. While uncommon, they are relatively specific for infective endocarditis. Janeway lesions, even less common, consist of small erythematous or hemorrhagic nonpainful areas that usually occur on the palms of the hands or the soles of the feet. In a different context, peripheral emboli from prosthetic cardiac valves, left ventricular mural thrombi, or marantic endocarditis may announce themselves in the tips of the fingers and toes as small, tender, painful areas that suddenly become pallid or cyanotic.

The Skin. The appearance of the skin and of the mucous membranes is now elaborated upon in order to supplement the above discussion. Skin appearance is important in terms of color, texture, swelling (edema), and localized lesions. Evaluation of small focal skin lesions sometimes benefits considerably when a magnifying glass or, still better, an ophthalmoscope is used as a simple means of magnification.

Cyanosis, apart from fingers, toes, and mucous membranes (see above), is detected in areas where the skin is thin, such as the ears, the tip of the nose, and the soles of the feet in infants. The cardiac implications of jaundice include chronic passive congestion of the liver, hemolysis due to the microangiopathic anemia of prosthetic cardiac valves, and the jaundice due to transient hemolysis following a large pulmonary infarct. Brawny induration of the legs and feet is a common consequence of peripheral edema in patients with chronic congestive heart failure. The bronze pigmentation of primary hemochromatosis is most prominent on exposed skin surfaces and is diagnostically important because of coexisting restrictive or dilated cardiomyopathy which is potentially reversible by phlebotomy.[27] Café au lait spots, freckles (especially axillary), and neurofibromas (skin-colored pedunculated tumors and subcutaneous nodules) (Fig. 2–30) are features of von Recklinghausen's disease that may be accompanied by pheochromocytoma. Symmetric vitiligo, especially of the distal extremities, arouses suspicion of Graves' disease (see above). In myxedema (see above), it is the **texture** of the skin that is important—coarse, thick, dry, with hair that is brittle, sparse, coarse, and without

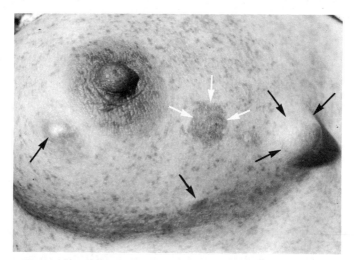

FIGURE 2–30. Café au lait spot *(white arrows)*, freckling, and cutaneous neurofibromas *(black arrows)* in a 38-year-old woman with von Recklinghausen's disease.

curl. In Ehlers-Danlos syndrome[3] (see above), the texture of the skin is striking and exhibits remarkable hyperextensibility, with a rubber-like response to stretch and cigarette-paper scars that result from fragility and poor healing. In pseudoxanthoma elasticum[3] (see above), the skin of the neck and axillae is reticular and telangiectatic with small tannish yellow papules that create the texture and appearance of a plucked chicken.

Subcutaneous **edema** is a time-honored hallmark of congestive heart failure. The edema is typically pitting and dependent, involving the ankles and feet in the upright position and the sacrum in the supine position. Facial edema (especially periorbital) occurs in recumbent infants with congestive heart failure unless the baby is put into an infant seat so its trunk is elevated. Localized *nonpitting* pretibial edema is related to hyperthyroidism (see above) and not to congestive heart failure.

A therapeutically important form of **discrete, localized skin lesion** in cardiac patients is acne. The most common location is the face, less commonly the shoulders or back. Acne puts susceptible patients at risk of staphylococcic infective endocarditis, so detection of these lesions sets the stage for advice on prophylactic skin care. Localized skin lesions may raise suspicion of coronary artery disease. Striated xanthomas (yellowish streaks) along the palmar creases (Fig. 2–31) are caused by type III (broad beta) hyperlipoproteinemia. Xanthomas (soft, yellowish plaques at the inner canthus of the eyelids) were mentioned earlier. Tuberous xanthomas are yellowish, coalescing nodules most commonly found on the elbows or knees. Eruptive xanthomas are crops of yellow-orange papules surrounded by erythematous halos, generally on the arms, legs, and buttocks.

In systemic amyloidosis, discrete localized cutaneous lesions may take the form of subtle, small, translucent, waxy, flat-top nodules. An ophthalmoscope or hand lens is especially useful in identifying these small lesions, which are ideal for punch biopsy.

Axillary freckling—Crowe's sign—is believed to be a useful diagnostic aid in von Recklinghausen's neurofibromatosis[28] (see above). Large widespread freckling or

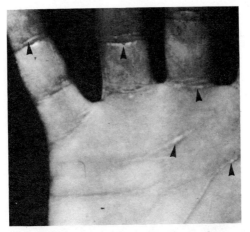

FIGURE 2–31. Striated xanthomas (yellowish streaks, *arrows*) along palmar creases in type III (broad beta) hyperliproteinemia.

lentiginosis (leopard syndrome) is sometimes associated with hypertrophic cardiomyopathy, especially when the lentigines are present from the first year of life.[29]

Localized linear scars along the course of veins, usually anticubital, imply "mainline" intravenous drug abuse (Fig. 2–32) with the risk of staphylococcic bacteremia and right-sided infective endocarditis. A small localized cutaneous scar may be the only visible remnant of the entrance site of the penetrating injury responsible for an acquired systemic arteriovenous fistula.

In acute rheumatic fever, subcutaneous nodules tend to localize over bony prominences of the elbows, dorsa of the hands or feet, and the malleoli or vertebrae. These nodules vary from pinhead to 1 to 2 cm and are subcutaneous (i.e., unattached to the skin) so that the integument moves freely over them.

In tuberous sclerosis, the cutaneous lesions are yellow to orange-red nevi varying in size from a few millimeters to a centimeter, symmetrically distributed on the malar and nasal skin. The lesions are also called adenoma sebaceum and are sometimes accompanied by cardiac rhabdomyoma.

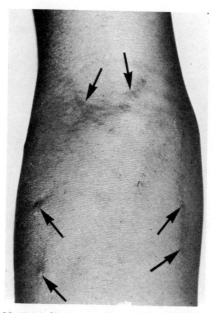

FIGURE 2–32. "Mainline" scars *(arrows)* along the tracts of arm veins in a 21-year-old female heroin addict with pulmonary valve infective endocarditis.

Muscles and Tendons. Abnormal appearance of **skeletal muscles** generally implies a decrease in mass (atrophy, dystrophy, wasting). A decrease in muscle mass can be relatively generalized as a result of the catabolic effects of chronic congestive heart failure. When these catabolic effects occur in infants and young children, the muscle wasting is accompanied by retardation of growth. Alternatively, the decrease in muscle mass may be highly selective, representing diagnostically specific phenotypic features of certain systemic neuromuscular diseases. An example of selective (regional) muscle wasting (dystrophy, atrophy) is myotonic muscular dystrophy (see Fig. 2–7) with involvement of superficial facial, temporalis, and sternocleidomastoid muscles, distal muscles of the forearms, and dorsiflexors of the feet. Cardiac involvement targets principally the specialized conduction tissues with abnormalities of impulse and conduction, as mentioned earlier.

The converse of muscle wasting is represented by "pseudohypertrophy," especially but not only of the calves, in boys with classic X-linked Duchenne muscular dystrophy (see Fig. 2–4*B*). Cardiac involvement is common and highly specific (see above).

As a rule, muscle weakness accompanies a *loss* of muscle mass, but occasionally flaccidity occurs *without* muscle wasting. A common example is the hypotonia of infants with Down syndrome[5] (Fig. 2–33). The hypotonia becomes less apparent or disappears altogether as the child grows older.

Examination of **tendons** can be diagnostically useful, with abnormalities varying from subtle to obvious. The Achilles tendons should be palpated routinely in adults in search of the thickening caused by tendon xanthomas which, when large and nodular, are apparent at a glance (Fig. 2–34). The diagnostic implication is coronary artery disease. Xanthomas attached to dorsal tendons of the hands may be invisible unless the fingers are gently and rhythmically flexed, imparting motion to the xanthomas that are attached to the tendons but not to the skin. Shortening of Achilles tendons is an important abnor-

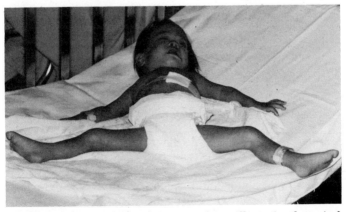

FIGURE 2–33. Young child with Down syndrome illustrating the typical hypotonic legs and hyperflexible hips. The bandage is postoperative.

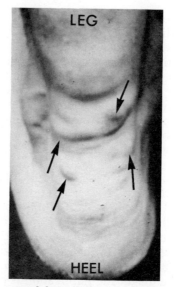

FIGURE 2–34. Large, nodular Achilles tendon xanthomas *(arrows)* in a young adult male with heterozygous familial hypercholesterolemia.

mality in boys with Duchenne muscular dystrophy (see Fig. 2–4*B*), causing them to walk on their toes, compromising an already tenuous balance.

The Thorax. The diagnostic usefulness of the appearance of the thorax lies in its general configuration and in regional abnormalities of bone or of soft tissue. The normal and abnormal movements of the thorax—patterns during active respiration—are dealt with in Chapter 7.

One of the most common clinical abnormalities of general thoracic appearance is the result of pulmonary emphysema (chronic obstructive lung disease). Richard C. Cabot's description of large-lunged emphysema suffices[31] (Fig. 2–35). "The diagnosis can usually be made by inspection alone. In typical cases the antero-posterior dimension of the chest is greatly increased, the interspaces are widened, and the costal angle is blunted, while the angle of Ludwig (formed by the junction of the manubrium with the second piece of the sternum) be-

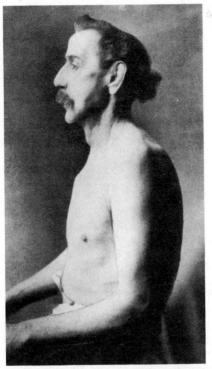

FIGURE 2–35. Barrel chest due to what Richard C. Cabot referred to as "large-lunged emphysema." (Reproduced from Cabot RC: Physical Diagnosis. New York, William Wood and Co, 1915. Courtesy of Dr. Sherman M. Mellinkoff, UCLA Medical Center.)

comes prominent. The shoulders are high and stooping and the neck is short."

Structural abnormalities of the thoracic spine and/or sternum vary from marked general distortions of thoracic configuration that are obvious at a glance to subtle abnormalities that reveal themselves only to pointed search. Kyphoscoliosis and pectus excavatum and carinatum are well-known features of the Marfan syndrome (Fig. 2–36A) (see above). Simple, innocent loss of thoracic kyphosis (straight back) is best sought with the patient sitting bolt upright and varies from mild to relatively

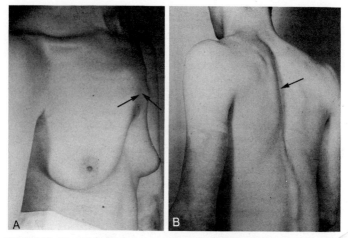

FIGURE 2–36. *A,* Marked pectus carinatum *(arrows)* in a young woman with the Marfan syndrome. *B,* Absence of normal thoracic vertebral lordosis (straight back, *arrows*) in an otherwise normal young man.

obvious (Fig. 2–36*B*). The accompanying decrease in anteroposterior chest dimensions results in physical signs that are sometimes mistaken for organic heart disease—a left parasternal systolic impulse and a pulmonic midsystolic murmur, for example. Importantly, this form of straight thoracic spine leaves the vertebrae mobile, in contrast to ankylosing spondylitis in which the appearance of the thorax is characterized by a rigid spine fused in flexion and in which coexisting aortic regurgitation is not uncommon. Pectus excavatum of moderate degree is easily overlooked in females with well-developed breasts. Marked pectus excavatum shifts the heart to the left and sometimes results in a parasternal systolic impulse and a pulmonic midsystolic murmur, signs similar to those described above in patients with a decrease in anteroposterior chest dimension due to loss of thoracic kyphosis.

Minor degrees of scoliosis are often identified during the bedside examination, but more likely in anteroposterior chest radiographs of otherwise normal people. This common form of scoliosis is almost always with the convexity to the *right*. Convexity to the *left* arouses suspicion of a systemic neuromuscular disease or polio-myelitis.

Abnormalities of thoracic configuration are relatively frequent in patients with congenital heart disease, but the hypothesis that these alterations are due to an increase in right ventricular mass alone is open to question.[32] The usual variety of chest deformity in such patients is anterior asymmetry, especially a left precordial bulge. When cardiac dyspnea in infants and young children causes repetitive traction on the diaphragmatic insertions of the rib cage during growth and development, nonrachitic Harrison's grooves commonly result.

Soft tissue abnormalities of the thorax are often diagnostically important. A case in point is the scar of a previous thoracotomy. A midline sternotomy scar is not likely to be overlooked, but lateral thoracotomy scars sometimes are. A lateral thoracotomy scar together with *ipsilateral* absence of the brachial arterial pulse is a feature of a shunt operation employing the subclavian artery on that side. A *left* thoracotomy scar together with

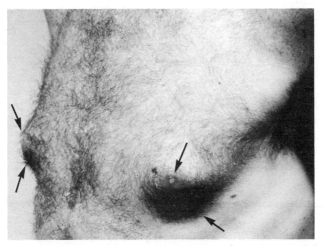

FIGURE 2–37. Bilateral gynecomastia in a male patient receiving digitalis glycosides in average maintenance doses.

absence of the *left* brachial pulse is a presumptive sign of a right aortic arch, generally with Fallot's tetralogy.

Abnormalities of the breasts occasionally take the form of male gynecomastia, unilateral or bilateral, in patients receiving digitalis glycosides[33] (Fig. 2–37). Female *hypomastia* is sometimes part of the asthenic habitus found in patients with mitral valve prolapse. In the 45 XO Turner syndrome, widely spaced nipples result from the broad shield chest (see Fig. 2–2A).

Physical appearance of the abdomen—see Chapter 8.

REFERENCES

1. Gombrich, E. H.: Meditations on a Hobby Horse. London, Phaidon, 1978.
2. Shakespeare, W.: King Henry V, Act II, Scene III.
3. McKusick, V. A.: Heritable Disorders of Connective Tissue. 4th ed. St. Louis, C. V. Mosby Company, 1972.
4. Farquhar, J. W.: The child of the diabetic woman. Arch. Dis. Childhood. 34:76, 1958.
5. Perloff, J. K.: The Clinical Recognition of Congenital Heart Disease. 3rd ed. Philadelphia, W. B. Saunders Company, 1987.
6. Burwell, C. S., Robin, E. D., Whaley, R. D., and Bickelmann, A. G.: Extreme obesity associated with alveolar hypoventilation—A pickwickian syndrome. Am. J. Med. 21:811, 1956.
7. Mackenzie, J.: Principles of Diagnosis and Treatment in Heart Affections. London, Oxford University Press, 1916.
8. Shakespeare, W.: King Richard III, Act III, Scene IV.
9. Perloff, J. K., and Phelps, E. T.: A review of Werner's syndrome, with a report of the second autopsied case. Ann. Intern. Med. 48:205, 1958.
10. Renteria, V. G., Ferrans, V. J., and Roberts, W. C.: The heart in the Hurler syndrome: Gross, histologic and ultrastructural observations in five necropsy cases. Am. J. Cardiol. 38:487, 1976.
11. Clarren, S. K., and Smith, D. W.: The fetal alcohol syndrome. N. Engl. J. Med. 298:1063, 1978.
12. Cayler, G. G., Blumenfeld, C. M., and Anderson, R. L.: Further studies of patients with the cardiofacial syndrome. Chest 60:161, 1971.
13. Roberts, N. K., Perloff, J. K., and Kark, R. A. P.: Cardiac conduction in the Kearns-Sayre syndrome (a neuromuscular disorder associated with progressive external ophthalmoplegia and pigmentary retinopathy). Am. J. Cardiol. 44:1396, 1979.
14. Silverman, K. H., Hutchins, G. M., and Bulkley, B. H.: Cardiac sarcoid: A clinicopathologic study of 84 unselected patients with systemic sarcoidosis. Circulation 58:1204, 1978.

15. Ruppert, G. B., Lindsay, J., and Barth, W. F.: Cardiac conduction abnormalities in Reiter's syndrome. Am. J. Med. 73:335, 1982.

16. Criscitiello, M. G., Ronan, J. A., Besterman, E. M., and Schoenwetter, W.: Cardiovascular abnormalities in osteogenesis imperfecta. Circulation 31:255, 1965.

17. Freedom, R. M., and Gerald, P. S.: Congenital heart disease and the "cat eye" syndrome. Am. J. Dis. Child. 126:16, 1973.

18. Heggtveit, H. A.: Syphilitic aortitis. A clinicopathologic autopsy study of 100 cases, 1950 to 1960. Circulation 29:346, 1964.

19. Editorial: Pulmonary arteriovenous fistula in hereditary hemorrhagic telangiectasia. Lancet 1:158, 1960.

20. Jeresatz, R. M., Husyar, R. J., and Basu, S.: Pierre Robin syndrome. Am. J. Dis. Child. 117:710, 1969.

21. Beaven, D. W., and Brooks, S. E.: A Color Atlas of the Nail in Clinical Diagnosis. Weert, Netherlands, Wolfe Medical Publications Ltd., 1984.

22. Edeiken, J.: Shoulder-hand syndrome following myocardial infarction with special reference to prognosis. Circulation 16:14, 1957.

23. Bittl, J. A., and Perloff, J. K.: Chronic post-rheumatic fever arthropathy of Jaccoud. Am. Heart J. 105:515, 1983.

24. Gellis, S. S., and Feingold, M.: Rubinstein-Taybi syndrome. Am. J. Dis. Child. 121:327, 1971.

25. Holt, M., and Oram, S.: Familial heart disease with skeletal malformation. Br. Heart J. 22:236, 1960.

26. Child, J. S., Perloff, J. K., Bach, P. M., Wolfe, A. D., Perlman, S., and Kark, R. A. P.: Cardiac involvement in Friedreich's ataxia. J. Am. Coll. Cardiol. 7:1370, 1986.

27. Dabestani, A., Child, J. S., Henze, E., Perloff, J. K., Schon, H., Figueroa, W. G., Schelbert, H. R., and Thessomboon, S.: Primary hemochromatosis: Anatomic and physiologic characteristics of the cardiac ventricles and their responses to phlebotomy. Am. J. Cardiol. 54:153, 1984.

28. Crowe, F. W.: Axillary freckling as a diagnostic aid in neurofibromatosis. Ann. Intern. Med. 61:1142, 1964.

29. Somerville, J., and Bonham-Carter, R. E.: The heart in lentiginosis. Br. Heart J. 34:58, 1972.

30. Perloff, J. K.: Neurological disorders and heart disease. In Braunwald, E. (ed): Heart Disease. 3rd ed. Philadelphia, W. B. Saunders Company, 1988.

31. Cabot, R. C.: Physical Diagnosis. New York, William Wood and Co., 1915.

32. Maxwell, G. M.: Chest deformity in children with congenital heart disease. Am. Heart J. 54:368, 1957.

33. LeWinn, E. B.: Gynecomastia during digitalis therapy. N. Engl. J. Med. 248:316, 1953.

THE ARTERIAL PULSE

"With careful practice, the trained finger can become a most sensitive instrument in the examination of the pulse."[1] Mackenzie trained his palpating finger by meticulous comparison with instrumental documentation from his polygraph (Fig. 3–1). The ancient art of feeling the pulse[2] (Fig. 3–2) can be applied in contemporary context to considerable diagnostic advantage. "In examining the pulse, our object is to obtain the most complete and exact knowledge attainable as to the circulation and to interpret accurately the facts we observe; the method to be followed must therefore be carefully described."[3] The purpose of this chapter is to describe carefully the methods of examining the arterial pulse and to call attention to the clinical advantages so derived.

The term "examination" refers to palpation, observation, and auscultation of arterial pulses. Certain pulses are examined routinely, others optionally depending in part upon the patient's age. Routine **palpation** in infants deals with the brachial and femoral arteries. In children and young adults, the important additional pulse is the carotid, whereas in older adults, routine palpation includes the carotids, brachials, radials, femorals, dorsalis pedis, posterior tibials, and the abdominal aorta. Selective palpation of other arterial pulses is performed chiefly but not exclusively in older adults and includes the subclavian, popliteal, ulnar, and digital (fingertip) pulses. **Observation** refers to visible arterial pulsations. Certain visible pulses are relatively obvious, such as the carotid pulsations of free aortic regurgitation or the serpentine brachial pulse of Monckeberg's sclerosis. Others are less obvious (and less important) and are overlooked unless specifically sought. An example is the pulsating dorsalis pedis in an infant with a large left-to-right shunt patent ductus arteriosus. Routine **auscultation** of arterial pulses depends chiefly upon the patient's age. In children and young adults, normal supraclavicular systolic murmurs are sought by placing the bell of the stethoscope over the subclavian arteries in the supraclavicular fossae. In older adults, auscultation of the carotids, subclavians, and femoral arteries should be routine. *Selective auscultation* is appropriate over the spine between the scapulae in patients with coarctation of the aorta. Selective auscultation over the abdominal aorta and its bifurcation and over the renal arteries is appropriate in some patients, especially older adults.

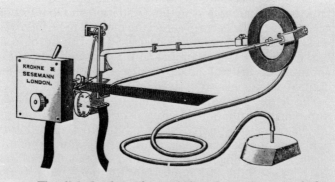

The clinical polygraph, consisting of a tambour attached to a Dudgeon's sphygmograph.

FIGURE 3–1. "This apparatus, which I have called the clinical polygraph, can be used for taking ... tracings of the radial pulse, with tracings of the apex beat, carotid, venous, or liver pulse ... ." (From Mackenzie J: Diseases of the Heart. London, Oxford University Press, 1908.)

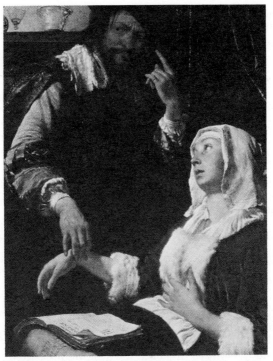

FIGURE 3–2. Franz van Mieris, "The Doctor's Visit." Kunsthistorisches Museum, Vienna. In female patients, decorum precluded palpation of any pulse except the radial.

INFORMATION DERIVED FROM THE ARTERIAL PULSE

"The point first to be noted is the frequency—the number of beats per minute—the regularity or irregularity of the beats as to time, and their equality or inequality in force. . . . We should naturally wish, in the next place, to estimate the force or strength of the pulse. . . . An important point to be investigated is the degree of constant pressure prevailing in the arteries. . . . The character of the beat is another matter for study; and brief as is the period occupied by it, each pulse wave presents a rise, duration, and fall."[3] These points were made by W. H. Broadbent in 1890. They are valid today and are addressed in this chapter.

A Systematic Approach

Examination of the arterial pulse must be systematic to avoid oversights. I recommend using a consistent sequence of evaluation, although that sequence need not be the same from examiner to examiner. The sequence used in this chapter is listed in Table 3–1.

Blood Pressure. Before the introduction of sphygmomanometry, Mackenzie stated, "The trained finger is as yet the best guide we have in judging the pressure in an artery. The fingertips become so educated in the course of time, that we readily appreciate the sensation conveyed in compressing an artery."[1] Systolic arterial pressure can be estimated by the amount of brachial arterial compression required to obliterate the ipsilateral radial pulse palpated by the examiner's other hand. When relatively mild brachial arterial compression in adults obliterates the radial arterial pulse, the systolic pressure is generally less than 120 mm Hg. When considerable compression is required to achieve this end, the systolic pressure usually exceeds 160 mm Hg.

Indirect measurement of blood pressure using an occluding cuff and the auscultatory technique was one of the earliest quantitative measurements of major importance applied at the bedside during the physical examination of the heart and circulation. Potain (1845–1901) introduced the sphygmomanometer.[4] The occluding cuff

TABLE 3–1. Examination of the Arterial Pulse

1. Blood pressure
2. Cardiac rate and rhythm
3. Wave form
4. Differential pulsations:
   a. Right/left, upper/lower
   b. Selective diminution, absence, or augmentation
5. Arterial thrills and murmurs
6. Structural properties

was developed almost simultaneously by Hill and Barnard in England and Riva-Rocci (Potain's pupil) in Italy.[4] However, for practical clinical use, a supplement to these two devices was required, namely, a reliable yet simple method for measuring blood pressure at the bedside. A pivotal figure in filling this need was the young Russian surgeon Nikolai Korotkoff, who wrote in 1905, "Immediately below a completely compressed artery (with obliteration of the lumen) no sounds are heard. As soon as the first drops of blood escape from under the site of pressure, we hear a clapping sound very distinctly. This sound is heard when the compressed artery is released and even before the appearance of pulsation in the peripheral branches."[5, 6] The next step was the binaural stethoscope, which facilitated detection of Korotkoff sounds over the brachial artery. The modern binaural stethoscope and the mercury or anaeroid cuff provide contemporary clinicians with a refined bedside method for the determination of systemic arterial pressure. The stethoscope should be well crafted and equipped with bell and diaphragm. The sphygmomanometer's compression cuff, the hand-operated rubber bulb for inflation, and the adjustable valve for cuff deflation have to be in perfect working order. The inflatable rubber bladder must be completely and securely contained within the sealed inelastic cuff so that even pressure is exerted over the area to which it is applied. Standard portable anaeroid manometers should be recalibrated periodically against a mercury manometer.

Taking the blood pressure is routine, but errors abound because of faulty technique, a conclusion difficult to escape when we observe those around us perform this common measurement. In addition to the instruments that must be in perfect working order (see above), correct cuff size is mandatory because an undersized cuff causes falsely high readings and an oversized cuff causes falsely low readings. Cuff size refers to the width and length of the inner inflatable rubber bladder, not to the cloth covering. Selection of appropriate cuff size is determined by the circumference of the limb, not the age of the patient. The width of the inflatable bladder should be approximately 40 per cent of the circumference of the midpoint of the limb to which the cuff is applied, and the length of the bladder within the cuff must completely encircle the extremity without overlapping.

Brachial arterial pressure should be taken in a quiet setting with the patient lying comfortably supine and the arms extended and relaxed parallel to and level with the thorax. Although upper extremity blood pressure in infants and adults is routinely determined with the patient in the horizontal supine position, a comfortable sitting position is an acceptable alternative in a young child, who may be more relaxed when sitting on the parent's lap. Sufficient time must be allowed to elapse for the patient to recover from recent activity or apprehension, especially in an outpatient setting. The blood pressure should be taken in both arms, because the systolic pressure tends to be somewhat higher in the right arm (as much as 15 mm Hg in adults). It is useful to palpate the brachial artery during cuff inflation to be certain that the inflation pressure is 20 to 30 mm Hg above the pressure required to obliterate the brachial pulse. The adjustable screw valve permits controlled, slow deflation of the cuff. Peak systolic pressure is identified by the appearance of clear Korotkoff sounds for two or more consecutive beats. Continued slow cuff deflation then determines the diastolic pressure, which is taken as the point at which Korotkoff sounds vanish rather than at the point of muffling, because the disappearance point is closer to the intra-arterial diastolic pressure. Inappropriately slow cuff deflation should be avoided; the accompanying venous congestion decreases the intensity of Korotkoff sounds, so that systolic pressure is underestimated while diastolic pressure is overestimated. Once the diastolic pressure is established, the cuff is deflated rapidly. At least 1 minute should elapse before blood pressure measurements are repeated in the same limb. Audibility of brachial arterial Korotkoff sounds is improved by having the patient open and close the fist vigorously a dozen or so times.

An "auscultatory gap" occasionally separates the initial audibility of Korotkoff sounds from their later audibility at a lower pressure. The importance of the auscultatory gap lies in misjudging systolic pressure when the cuff is inflated to a level within the gap itself. This error is avoided by inflating the cuff well above the level necessary to obliterate the palpable brachial arterial pulse (see above). In addition to using palpation to avoid the misleading auscultatory gap, the seemingly outmoded technique of palpation for estimating arterial pressure occasionally serves a useful purpose in modern acute care bedside medicine. When Korotkoff sounds are indistinct or inaudible, systolic and diastolic pressures can be estimated by palpation in the following manner. After standard cuff inflation, the approximate peak systolic pressure is the level at which a palpable brachial pulse first consistently reappears when the cuff is slowly deflated. The diastolic pressure is then estimated by detecting a distinctive snapping quality of the palpable pulse as the cuff is deflated further.

There is a prevailing misconception about the inaccuracy of determinations of cuff brachial arterial pressure in patients with obese arms. Error is averted by selecting a cuff of appropriate size, i.e., width and length of the inner inflatable bladder as recommended above. Recall that the circumference of the limb is the factor that determines appropriate cuff size. A cuff of proper width (40 per cent of the circumference of the midpoint of the limb) should completely encircle the arm and exert an even pressure over the enclosed area.

A variation on the usefulness of brachial arterial blood pressure is the "proportional pulse pressure" calculated as the difference between systolic and diastolic blood pressures divided by the systolic blood pressure. A proportional pulse pressure of 25 per cent or less identifies about 90 per cent of patients with left ventricular failure and cardiac indices of 2.2 L/min/m^2 or less.

If the only available cuff does not adequately encircle the arm, the same cuff might be tried on the forearm while the bell of the stethoscope is applied to the radial artery for the detection of Korotkoff sounds (Fig. 3–3A). This technique is satisfactory provided that the forearm is relatively uniform in circumference (cylindrical), but not when a conical forearm prevents an even distribution

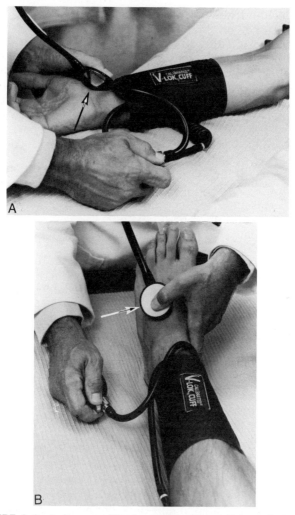

FIGURE 3–3. *A,* Forearm blood pressure. The cuff is applied to a relatively cylindrical (not conical) forearm. The bell of the stethoscope *(arrow)* is placed over the radial artery for detection of Korotkoff sounds. *B,* Calf blood pressure. If a proper size leg cuff is not readily available, a standard arm cuff can be applied to the distal calf. Korotkoff sounds are sought by placing the *bell* of the stethoscope *(arrow)* over the dorsalis pedis (shown here) or posterior tibial artery, the latter generally providing a better skin seal.

of pressure over the encircled area. Properly determined forearm blood pressure is a reasonable approximation of brachial arterial pressure.

In adults, especially those beyond middle age, **orthostatic hypotension** can be identified by recording brachial arterial pressure in the supine and upright positions (standing or with legs dangling over the edge of the examining table or bed). Assumption of the upright position is normally accompanied by no more than a 5 to 15 mm Hg decline in systolic pressure, whereas diastolic pressure tends to rise. These changes are associated with slight reflex tachycardia. A special form of postural hypotension is provoked by assumption of the left lateral decubitus position.[7] To elicit left lateral decubitus hypotension, the blood pressure cuffs should first be placed on both arms and blood pressure recorded in the supine position, bearing in mind that in some normal adults, right arm pressure exceeds left arm pressure (see above). The patient is then asked to turn into the *right* lateral decubitus position while blood pressure is taken in the *left* arm. After a brief return to the supine position, the patient is asked to turn into the *left* lateral decubitus position while blood pressure is recorded from the *right* arm. Normally, there is no difference from supine to either right or left lateral decubitus position. Left lateral decubitus hypotension consists of a fall in both systolic *and* diastolic pressure, sometimes accompanied by dyspnea, palpitations, weakness, and lightheadedness.[7]

When infants are quieted with a bottle or pacifier, it is possible to obtain blood pressure by the cuff and auscultatory method, as described above. Alternatively, the "flush" blood pressure method can be used. An uninflated cuff is applied to the infant's forearm, which is elevated while the limb distal to the cuff is gently massaged to induce blanching. The cuff is then inflated above anticipated systolic pressure while the arm remains elevated and blanched. The arm is then lowered to the horizontal position while the cuff is slowly deflated. The point at which the blanched hand becomes flushed is an estimate of the *mean* arterial pressure. The flush method has shortcomings, requiring at least two persons to perform the task, and even then only a mean arterial pressure is secured. A convenient, simple bedside Doppler device can be used by a single observer to record systolic *and* diastolic pressures.

Lower extremity blood pressure from the popliteal artery is best determined with the patient prone. Whether this procedure is employed depends upon the degree of clinical suspicion, which is generally based upon prior palpation of upper and lower extremity arterial pulses (see below). A cuff of appropriate size is carefully applied to the thigh. The popliteal artery is then identified by palpation. The thigh cuff is inflated to a level just above the brachial arterial systolic pressure. It is important to inflate *slowly* to avoid discomfort, if not pain, induced by rapid thigh compression. Systolic and diastolic pressures are estimated by auscultation of popliteal arterial Korotkoff sounds. Not uncommonly, only systolic Korotkoff sounds are clearly heard, but this is not a shortcoming in the assessment of differential blood pressure in coarctation of the aorta, for example, because diagnostic differences in arm and leg pressures are based upon *systolic*, not diastolic levels. The *auscultatory* systolic pressure in the leg is normally about 10 mm Hg higher than the *intra-arterial* measurement, but the diastolic pressures are the same.

If the above technique for determining lower extremity blood pressure proves unsatisfactory, the patient can be returned to the supine position, and a cuff of appropriate size (often an arm cuff) is applied to the lower half of the calf (Fig. 3–3*B*). Korotkoff sounds are then sought by placing the bell of the stethoscope over the dorsalis pedis or preferably the posterior tibial artery after their pulses have been identified by palpation. The disadvantage of this method is that it cannot be used in infants, and Korotkoff sounds are at best inconsistently heard over the dorsalis pedis or posterior tibial arteries in older patients, even when those arteries are normal and pulsatile. Exercising the limb sometimes increases audibility of Korotkoff sounds over the pedal pulses and over the popliteal artery.

Cardiac Rate and Rhythm. "The point first to be noted

is the frequency—the number of beats per minute—the regularity or irregularity of the beats as to time, and their equality or inequality in force. This is simple and easy."[3] Heart rate is routinely determined by palpating an arterial pulse, although cardiac auscultation is sometimes employed for this purpose (see below). Accurate estimates of rate are now taken for granted, requiring nothing more than a palpable artery and a watch with a second hand. However, an appropriate watch was long in coming as a part of the clinician's bedside accouterments (see Chapter 1).

Counting the pulse should proceed for at least 30 seconds, but when the rhythm is irregular, a full minute provides a more accurate basis for judgment. Under certain circumstances—atrial fibrillation or marked pulsus alternans, for example—the palpable arterial pulse is slower than the rate of ventricular contraction. This "pulse deficit" is identified by comparing the rate of the palpable arterial pulse with the heart rate as judged by simultaneous precordial auscultation.

It goes without saying that the normal cardiac rate varies with age, from person to person, and under different circumstances in the same person. In 1890, Broadbent wrote:[3]

> The average frequency of the pulse in the adult male is 72 beats per minute; in the female about 80; in the child it is much more frequent, and it gradually loses in frequency from infancy onwards. There are slight diurnal variations . . . , but independently of any such influences, the pulse is more frequent in the evening than in the morning . . . , and it would appear from various considerations . . . that during a long night's sleep the circulation runs downs in vigour as well, and not only in frequency.

"There are no deviations from the normal character of the pulse so easy to recognize as irregularities in rhythm. . . ."[1] Mackenzie went on to divide cases into two groups, namely, those in which the duration of systole was *regular*, and those in which it was of *variable* duration. Characterization of arrhythmias based upon the arterial pulse is, with important exceptions, imprecise, but Mackenzie's grouping remains a useful point of departure. If the rhythm is irregular (variable duration of systole), it is necessary to establish whether the irregularity has a pattern. Simple atrial premature beats do not, as a rule, interrupt subsequent cycle lengths, provided that the sinus node recovery time is normal. Conversely, ventricular premature beats are typically followed by "compensatory pauses." In either case, it is usually apparent from the pulse that the basic rhythm is regular. A pronounced sinus arrhythmia sometimes clouds the issue and may lead to the mistaken conclusion that the basic rhythm is irregular. When circumstances permit, this error is avoided by determining the rhythm with the patient's breath held comfortably in the respiratory midposition, a maneuver that abolishes sinus arrhythmia that is coupled to respiration. Group beating generally means that the basic rhythm is regular but is systematically interrupted by recurrences of premature beats or cyclic absence of a beat. Complete loss of regular rhythm (variable duration of systole) is characteristic of atrial fibrillation. Even so, a *slow* ventricular response in atrial fibrillation may be accompanied by differences in cycle lengths that are too subtle to be detected by palpation of the arterial pulse. Multiple ventricular premature beats sometimes disturb the basic rhythm to a degree that precludes confidently distinguishing that arrhythmia from atrial fibrillation. Examination of the jugular venous pulse in this setting serves to clarify the issue (see Chapter 4).

The Valsalva maneuver, described in detail in Chapter 6, is mentioned here because of the associated changes in heart rate which are detectable at the bedside. Specifically, Phase 2 is accompanied by reflex tachycardia and a small pulse, while Phase 4 (overshoot) is accompanied by reflex bradycardia. In the presence of severe congestive heart failure, there is loss of the reflex tachycardia of Phase 2 and of the reflex bradycardia of Phase 4. Accordingly, determination of the pulse rate during Phases 2 and 4 of the Valsalva maneuver is a simple bedside method for assessing heart failure.

Wave Form. Analysis of wave form is one of the most important aspects of the examination of the arterial pulse. The stage is set by an appreciation of the wave form of the *normal* arterial pulse in healthy persons of all ages under varying conditions of relaxation and stress.

Assessment of wave form begins with selection of the pulse most appropriate for a given examination. The basis for this judgment depends in part upon the clinician's objective, upon the structural state or physical properties of the arterial wall, and upon the patient's age. Because a prime objective is to secure the most accurate representation of the central arterial pulse, it is well to remember a point made by Carl Wiggers:[8] "By the time the pulse wave reaches the radial artery, friction has modified the fundamental contour and in addition has wiped out all of the smaller oscillations which exist in the central pulse" (Fig. 3–4). The carotid arterial pulse is readily accessible to the palpating finger or thumb and provides a relatively close approximation of the wave form of the central aortic pulse. Before palpating the carotid, however, certain variables must be taken into account, such as atherosclerotic obstruction in adults, kinking of the right carotid (see below), the presence of a thrill or shudder, and in infants, a short neck that precludes use of carotid arterial palpation for routine assessment of wave form. Alternatively, certain wave forms are more obvious in *peripheral* pulses. Examples include pulsus alternans, which is best detected in radial and femoral arteries, and pulsus bisferiens, best detected in the brachial artery. However, these few constraints should not obscure the value of information derived from palpation of the carotid pulse in most older children and adults.

The **technique of palpation** is all-important. For practical purposes, it is best to begin the examination of arterial pulse wave form by palpating the brachial arteries, which are convenient and accessible from infancy through adulthood. It is most convenient for palpation to start with the right brachial pulse (Fig. 3–5). The examiner should be in a comfortable position that permits concentration and ready access to the brachial pulse without stooping or leaning forward. These points were emphasized by Mackenzie, who recommended that " . . . One's whole attention should be concentrated upon the observation."[1] Ancient Chinese physicians were enjoined to

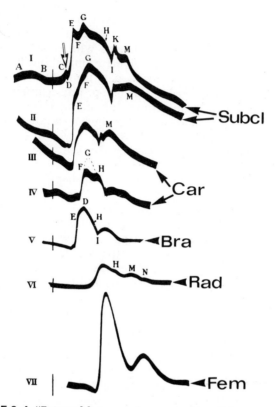

FIGURE 3–4. "Retraced human pulse curves from different arteries." The tracings show modification in contour from the central pulses (subclavian and carotid) to distal pulses (brachial, radial, femoral). Arrows and labels are my additions. (From Wiggers CJ: The Pressure Pulses in the Cardiovascular System. London, Longmans, Green and Co., 1928, p 77.)

banish all other thoughts from their minds in order to concentrate on the pulse.[2] Although these directives are excessive in modern context, it still holds true that without reasonable care and attention to arterial pulse wave form, oversights are bound to occur.

Routine palpation of the *right brachial pulse* is best accomplished with the thumb of the examiner's right

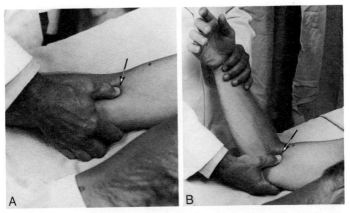

FIGURE 3–5. *A*, Palpation of the right brachial pulse with the thumb while the patient's arm lies at his or her side with the palm up. *B*, Palpation of the right brachial pulse with the patient's elbow resting in the palm of the examiner's hand. The thumb explores the antecubital fossa *(arrow)* while the patient's forearm is passively raised and lowered to achieve maximum relaxation of muscles around the elbow.

hand as the patient's arm lies supinated at his or her side (Fig. 3–5A). As the thumb explores the antecubital fossa for the brachial arterial pulse, the patient's elbow can rest in the palm of the examiner's right hand, while the free left hand passively raises and lowers the patient's forearm to achieve maximum relaxation of muscles around the antecubital fossa (Fig. 3–5B). In infants, gentle restraint of the right hand or wrist sometimes prevents undesirable movement of the arm, but forceful restraint must be avoided.

The ease with which palpation of the brachial pulse is achieved is influenced by the thickness and compressibility of the tissues between the examining finger and the artery and by the firmness of the tissue bed upon which the artery rests. Accordingly, a brachial artery is easier to palpate when it is relatively superficial and when resting upon a firm support. The pulse is difficult to palpate in an obese or muscular arm. Pulsatile, tortuous, thick-walled brachial arteries in older adults with Monckeberg's sclerosis (Fig. 3–6) may roll away when palpated, but

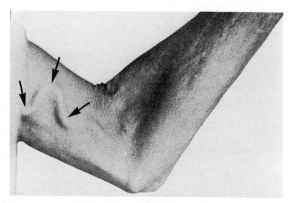

FIGURE 3–6. The thickened, serpentine brachial artery of Moncke-berg's sclerosis visible beneath the skin of the antecubital fossa *(arrows).* (From Cabot RC: Physical Diagnosis. New York, William Wood and Co, 1915. Courtesy of Dr. Sherman M. Mellinkoff, UCLA Medical Center.)

despite this difficulty, the thumb can almost always fix the serpentine brachial pulse against its bed.

Once the brachial artery is identified by the palpating thumb, progressive gentle pressure is exerted until the maximal systolic impact of the pulse is elicited. The examiner should then vary the pressure ever so slightly while forming a visual image of the components of the wave form (Fig. 3–7).

Palpation of the *carotid pulse* is accomplished with the examiner at the patient's right side. The right thumb is applied to the patient's left carotid artery (Fig. 3–8A) and then the left thumb is separately applied to the patient's right carotid (Fig. 3–8B). This technique permits comfortable application of the thumb without awkward bending of the wrist, a maneuver that decreases sensitivity in the fingertips. The thumb should gently and slowly exert pressure on the carotid pulse to elicit the maximal systolic impact as described above. In so doing, the artery should be palpated in the lower third of the neck to avoid inadvertent stimulation of the carotid sinus, especially in older adults.

Palpation of the *femoral arterial pulse* is achieved with

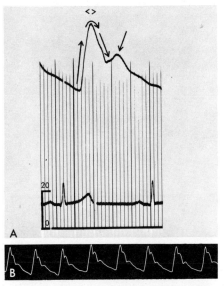

FIGURE 3–7. *A,* Normal intra-arterial brachial pulse showing the ascending limb, peak, descending limb, and dicrotic wave. *B,* Normal indirect radial pulse recorded by Mackenzie with his polygraph (see Fig. 3–1) applied to the wrist.

the examiner at the patient's right side while applying the right thumb to the left femoral artery (Fig. 3–9*A*) and then the left thumb to the right femoral artery (Fig. 3–9*B*). The pulse should be compressed gently and slowly as described above.

The *radial pulse* was the time-honored site for palpation when patients, especially women, were not disrobed for examination (see Fig. 3–2). Mackenzie gave impetus to use of the radial pulse because it was the most convenient site to which he could fix his polygraph (see Fig. 3–1). For routine assessment of wave form, however, the relatively altered contour of the radial pulse makes it of less value than the more central brachial and carotid pulses (see Fig. 3–4), except for detection of pulsus alternans (see below).

For radial pulse palpation, the patient's hand should be supinated and comfortably supported. The examiner's

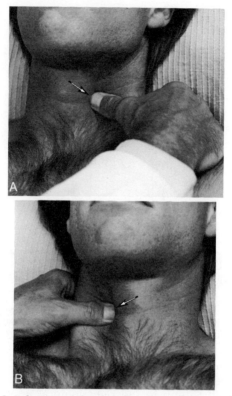

FIGURE 3–8. Palpation of the carotid pulse. *A*, The examiner places
the right thumb *(arrow)* on the patient's left carotid artery. *B*, The left
thumb *(arrow)* is then applied separately to the right carotid.

thumb (Fig. 3–10*A*) or the tip of a single finger, preferably
the index finger (Fig. 3–10*B*), is then applied to the pulse.
The index finger is slightly more sensitive than the thumb,
an observation used to advantage when palpating a relatively small pulse, such as the radial. The degree of
pressure applied to elicit the maximal systolic impact is
similar to that described above.

In infants, palpation of the radial pulse has inherent
limitations. "The infant's radial artery is naturally very
small. We are not conscious of its presence, being unable

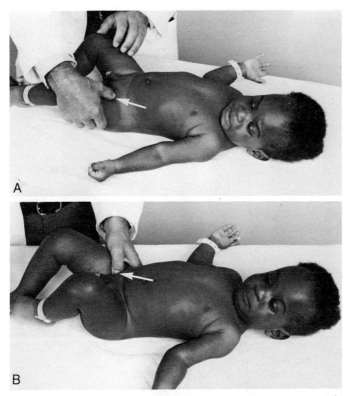

FIGURE 3–9. Palpation of the femoral pulse. *A*, The examiner's right thumb is applied to the patient's left femoral pulse *(arrow)* and then *(B)* the left thumb to the right femoral pulse *(arrow)*.

to differentiate it from the surrounding structures, and we only recognize its pulse when the finger presses the artery against the bone. This inability to feel the artery as a distinct structure is due not only to the smallness of the vessel, but to the fact that very often the padding of subcutaneous fat is relatively great in the very young."[1]

Recognition of abnormalities of wave form requires an understanding of the wave form of the **normal arterial pulse** (see Fig. 3–7), which varies according to physiologic state, patient age, and distance from the aortic root

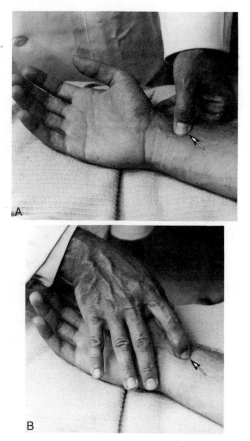

FIGURE 3–10. Palpation of the radial pulse. The thumb *(A)* or the index finger *(B)* is applied to the radial artery *(arrow).*

(see Fig. 3–4). Let us begin by characterizing the normal *brachial* arterial pulse from childhood to young adulthood. Specific attention is paid to the ascending limb, the peak, and the descending limb (see Fig. 3–7). With advancing age, a decrease in arterial distensibility (a more rigid arterial wall) results in a steeper rate of rise, a higher peak pressure, and a more rapid descent. Otherwise, the normal ascending limb rises smoothly to a single, somewhat rounded peak. The descending limb is less steep than the ascending and is interrupted by an incisura, i.e., a brief distinct downward displacement associated with closure of the aortic valve. The pulse wave then rises slightly (the dicrotic wave) before declining gradually throughout diastole. The incisura and the dicrotic wave of a normal pulse are not palpable. Nor is the slight shoulder (anacrotic notch) that is sometimes recorded on the ascending limb (see Fig. 3–4, subclavian pulse, upper left arrow).

Mackenzie's description of the normal arterial pulse is close if not identical to contemporary descriptions[1] (see Fig. 3–7B):

> There is first an abrupt rise, then a fall, followed by a continuation of the wave at about the same level. This period is usually described as being divided into two, the abrupt rise spoken of as the primary or percussion wave, and the latter portion as the tidal or pre-dicrotic wave. . . . With the closure of the aortic valve, the aortic pressure falls rapidly to the bottom of the aortic notch. . . . This fall is interrupted by a distinct rise in pressure, represented by the dicrotic wave.

For the purpose of this discussion, **abnormal arterial pulse** wave forms are designated as diminished (small, weak, hypokinetic with or without a sustained, delayed peak), increased (large, strong, hyperkinetic), and double-peaked (double systolic peak or systolic/diastolic peaks).

A *diminished arterial pulse* is perceived as a gentle impact. The palpating thumb or finger senses the gentle rate of rise. The peak remains relatively distinct but is reduced, ill-defined, and sometimes late. Depressed left ventricular systolic function is a case in point, resulting in a diminished, small, weak, hypokinetic arterial pulse with gentle ascending limb and a perceptible but reduced single peak. In severe aortic valve stenosis, the arterial pulse is also diminished, with a slow ascending limb (parvus), and a peak that is ill-defined and late (tardus) (Fig. 3–11A). Mackenzie wrote,[1] "When there is marked narrowing of the aortic orifice, the full effect of the ventricular systole upon the arterial column is not at once developed, as the aortic stenosis offers an increased resistance. Hence, the impact of the pulse wave on the

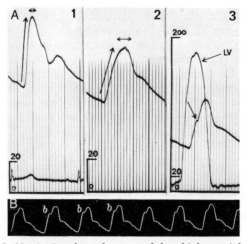

FIGURE 3–11. *A*, Panel 1, the normal brachial arterial pulse for comparison with Panel 2, the pulse in aortic valve stenosis, which illustrates the typical slow rate of rise and delayed, broad crest. Panel 3 shows simultaneous left ventricular (LV) and brachial arterial pulses of aortic stenosis with lower arrow pointing to a nonpalpable anacrotic notch. *B*, "Anacrotic pulse in a case of aortic stenosis" from Mackenzie.[1]

finger is not sudden, but feels to push against the finger in a somewhat leisurely fashion. The tracing in such a case represents a slanting of the stroke with an interruption near the top—an anacrotic-pulse tracing" (Fig. 3–11*B*). The anacrotic notch is seldom if ever palpable.

An *increased arterial pulse* can occur with single or double systolic peaks and with normal or wide pulse pressure (Figs. 3–12 and 3–13). The increased arterial pulse is sensed by the palpating thumb or finger as a conspicuously brisk impact (increased rate of rise). Whether the *rapid fall* after the systolic crest is sensed by palpation is open to question, but that may be so when the increased pulse is caused by pure severe aortic regurgitation (Fig. 3–13). The distinction between an increased arterial pulse with or without wide pulse pressure cannot always be established by palpation, but an attempt to do so can be made by determining the magnitude of brachial

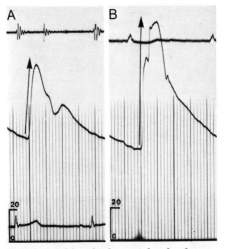

FIGURE 3–12. *A*, Normal brachial arterial pulse for comparison with *(B)* the brachial pulse in pure severe mitral regurgitation that exhibits a brisk rate of rise *(arrow)* with only a modest increase in pulse pressure.

arterial compression necessary to obliterate the simultaneously palpated radial pulse. An increased arterial pulse with *normal* pulse pressure requires no more than the normal amount of brachial compression to obliterate the radial pulse. When simultaneous brachial and radial palpation arouses suspicion of an *increase* in pulse pressure, it must then be determined whether the increased pulse pressure is due to *systolic* hypertension (older adult) or to systolic hypertension with low *diastolic* pressure, as in chronic severe aortic regurgitation (Fig. 3–13) or large left-to-right shunt through a patent ductus arteriosus (Fig. 3–14). When a wide pulse pressure is due to systolic hypertension (diminished arterial distensibility of old age), the rate of rise of the ascending limb is no more than moderately brisk. However, when the wide pulse pressure is due to high systolic pressure *and* low diastolic pressure in younger patients with distensible arterial walls, the rate of rise is not only brisk, but markedly so (Figs. 3–13 and 3–14).

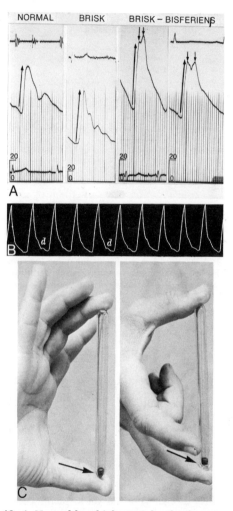

FIGURE 3–13. *A,* Normal brachial arterial pulse for comparison with brachial pulses in moderate to severe pure aortic regurgitation. The latter show a brisk single-peaked pulse and two brisk bisferiens pulses, one with unequal and the other with equal crests. *B,* "Pulse of extreme aortic regurgitation" (Mackenzie[1]). *C,* Toy water hammer consisting of a sealed glass tube containing mercury *(arrow)* in a vacuum. As the tube is quickly inverted, the mercury falls abruptly from one end to the other, imparting a jolt or impact to the thumb or fingertip.

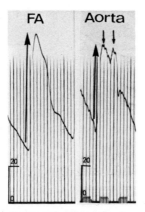

FIGURE 3–14. Femoral arterial (FA) pulse in an infant with large patent ductus arteriosus, showing a brisk rate of rise *(arrow)*, wide pulse pressure, and single peak. The central aortic pulse in the same patient is bisferiens *(double arrows)*.

The increased arterial pulse with wide pulse pressure of free aortic regurgitation has been compared to a water hammer, a term coined in 1844 by Thomas Watson, an English physician. The water hammer was a popular toy in Victorian England and consisted of a sealed glass tube containing water in a vacuum. Solids and liquids fall at the same rate in a vacuum, so when the glass tube is quickly inverted, the water column (or mercury column) falls abruptly from one end of the tube to the other (see Fig. 3–13C), and the fingertip holding the inverted end senses a sudden impact or jolt. The Victorian toy has long since vanished, but the term "water hammer" is still used to describe the arterial pulse of pure free aortic regurgitation. The "Corrigan pulse" of aortic regurgitation properly refers to a *visible*, not a palpable, pulse as described by Dominic J. Corrigan in 1832.[9]

When a patient affected by the disease is stripped, the arterial trunks of the head, neck and superior extremities immediately catch the eye by their singular pulsation. . . . From its singular and striking appearance, the name of *visible pulsation* is given to this beating of the arteries. . . . It is much more marked in the arteries of the head and neck in the erect than in the horizontal posture;

and a patient suffering under the disease himself, first points it out. . . .

Double-peaked pulses are of two types—those with two systolic peaks and those with one systolic and one diastolic peak. The term "double" is preferable to "twin peaking," because the latter designation implies that the two crests are similar, which is not necessarily the case (see Figs. 3–13*A* and 3–14). By convention, the double-peaked systolic pulse is designated "bisferiens," whereas a paired systolic/diastolic pulse is designated "dicrotic" (Fig. 3–15). The terms matter less than the clarity of the message, but it is not beside the point that, literally translated, "dicrotic" and "bisferiens" mean the same thing. "Dicrotic" has a Greek root: *di* = twice; *krotos* = beat. "Bisferiens" has a Latin root: *bis* = two; *ferire* = to beat.

"Anacrotic" is unimportant as a practical bedside designation for double-peaking of the systolic pulse because,

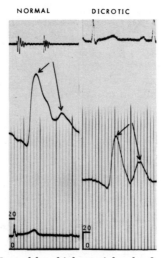

NORMAL   DICROTIC

FIGURE 3–15. Normal brachial arterial pulse for comparison with a dicrotic pulse that shows a single systolic crest *(first arrow)* and an amplified dicrotic wave *(second arrow)*.

as mentioned earlier, the anacrotic pulse is seldom palpable even when clearly recorded (see Fig. 3–11).

Double systolic peaks most commonly take the form of the bisferiens pulse of pure aortic regurgitation (see Fig. 3–13A). The two crests may be equal, or either the first or second crest can be the larger (see Figs. 3–13A and 3–14). The two peaks are not only palpable but are sometimes audible as double Korotkoff sounds heard as the blood pressure cuff is deflated. Double systolic peaks of the arterial pulse also occur with hypertrophic cardiomyopathy, generally obstructive (Fig. 3–16), but palpation usually detects only the brisk rise and sharp initial crest.

The designation "dicrotic pulse" is, by convention, applied when the second peak occurs during diastole (see Fig. 3–15). The amplified dicrotic wave is seldom palpable.

Pulsus alternans, originally described by Traube in 1872,[10] refers to alternation of the strength (force, impact) of the pulse sensed by palpation in the absence of arrhythmia or of a significant variation in interval between

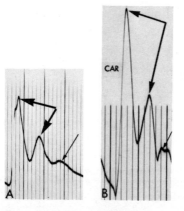

FIGURE 3–16. *A*, Direct brachial and *(B)* indirect carotid (CAR) arterial pulses in two patients with hypertrophic obstructive cardiomyopathy. The wave forms are similar, showing brisk rates of rise and double systolic peaks *(bold arrows)*. Thin arrow points to low-amplitude dicrotic waves, confirming the systolic timing of the two preceding crests.

beats (Fig. 3–17). Pulsus alternans can also be identified by beat-to-beat differences in the intensity of Korotkoff sounds (see below). Mechanical alternation of a systemic arterial pulse is a useful sign of depressed left ventricular systolic function. Alternate beats differ from each other in their peak systolic pressures, but what is probably sensed by palpation is the alternating rate of rise of the ascending limb (Fig. 3–17). Mechanical alternation is sometimes so marked that the weak beat is not perceived at all—"total mechanical alternans," effectively halving the cardiac rate as judged by the arterial pulse.

Mechanical alternans tends to become more prominent as the pulse wave moves peripherally. Accordingly, the radial and femoral pulses are usually more revealing than the carotids and brachials. Pulsus alternans is best elicited with the thumb applied to a femoral artery or the thumb or finger applied to a radial artery, gradually increasing compression until the impact of the pulse is maximal. As compression is slowly released, the examiner senses a decrease in impact of alternate beats. It is desirable to examine the pulse for alternation during quiet breathing or with the patient's breath held comfortably in the respiratory mid-position to avoid respiratory variations

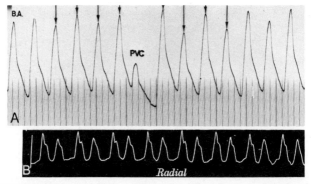

FIGURE 3–17. *A*, Brachial arterial (BA) pulse showing typical pulsus alternans *(vertical arrows)* exaggerated after a premature ventricular contraction (PVC). *B*, "Radial pulse showing the rhythmical irregularity (pulsus alternans)" (Mackenzie[1]). Note the beat-to-beat alternation in peak systolic pressure *and* in the rate of rise of the ascending limbs.

in the arterial pulse. When this maneuver is impractical because of dyspnea, the radial pulse should be palpated for alternation while the patient sits with the legs over the bedside or examining table. The latter maneuver, by decreasing venous return, tends to exaggerate alternation, and the upright position permits the patient to breathe more comfortably or even briefly to hold the breath. Nitroglycerin may serve the same purposes by decreasing venous return and relieving dyspnea. An important practical point is for the examiner to anticipate premature ventricular contractions because ventricular ectopic beats transiently provoke or exaggerate pulsus alternans, as shown in Figure 3–17A.

Pulsus alternans can also be detected by sphygmomanometry. The cuff pressure is slowly lowered from above systolic. Auscultation at the brachial artery initially detects Korotkoff sounds at half the ventricular rate. When the cuff pressure is lowered further, Korotkoff sounds are heard at a rate that suddenly doubles.

Pulsus alternans must be distinguished from the alternating strong/weak beats of a bigeminal pulse in which the weak beat is premature (Fig. 3–18). Traube drew a careful distinction between pulsus bigeminus and pulsus alternans.[10]

Pulsus paradoxus is a term that was introduced into clinical medicine by Adolph Kussmaul (1873) to describe the marked inspiratory fall in systemic arterial blood pressure in constrictive pericarditis.[11] The inspiratory decline is *not* really "paradoxical" but instead is an exaggeration of the normal inspiratory decrease in systolic pressure. What Kussmaul referred to, however, was a pulse that dropped markedly and unexpectedly, hence

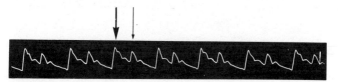

FIGURE 3–18. "Tracings of a bigeminal pulse" (Mackenzie[1]) (arrows mine) showing that the premature beat *(thin arrow)* is the weaker.

"paradoxically," with inspiration despite the fact that the heart rate and rhythm remained unchanged.

Normal inspiration in a healthy adult results in no more than a 3 to 4 mm Hg decline in systolic pressure. Even a relatively deep inspiration seldom causes a decline that reaches 10 mm Hg. Accordingly, the term "pulsus paradoxus" applies when the inspiratory decrease *exceeds* 10 mm Hg.

Pulsus paradoxus occurs in certain forms of cardiac disease and in certain forms of pulmonary disease. In the former, a paradoxical pulse is most frequently associated with pericardial tamponade, less commonly with chronic constrictive pericarditis which prompted Kussmaul's original description.[11] In both of these cardiac disorders, pulsus paradoxus is characterized by abnormal falls in systolic *and* diastolic pressures, reflecting an exaggerated inspiratory decline in left ventricular volume. The most common *noncardiac* cause of a paradoxical pulse is pulmonary emphysema (Fig. 3–19). The decrease in lung compliance magnifies the normal inspiratory decline in left ventricular volume and in the systolic and diastolic

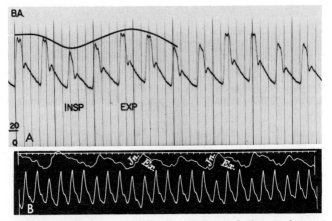

FIGURE 3–19. *A*, Pulsus paradoxus in an adult with chronic obstructive lung disease. Inspiration (INSP) is accompanied by a moderate fall in diastolic pressure, whereas expiration (EXP) results in an exaggerated rise in systolic pressure. *B*, Pulsus paradoxus "from a case of capillary bronchitis and catarrhal pneumonia" (Mackenzie[1]).

arterial pressures. Airway obstruction exaggerates the paradoxical pulse. Inspiration continues to cause an abnormal decline in systolic and diastolic pressures, while expiration is accompanied by an excessive *rise* in systolic pressure (above normal) (Fig. 3–19).

To elicit the paradoxical pulse, the patient should be comfortably positioned with the trunk raised to a level that minimizes respiratory excursions. The patient is then specifically instructed to breathe as regularly and quietly as comfort permits. The examiner's thumb is applied to the brachial arterial pulse with enough compression to elicit the maximal systolic impact. Compression is released gradually and in a stepwise fashion while the examiner observes the patient's respiratory movements by glancing at the chest or abdomen at each stepwise decrease in brachial arterial compression. As pressure on the brachial artery decreases, a level is reached at which the pulse diminishes or even vanishes altogether during inspiration.

The paradoxical pulse is even more readily detected with a sphygmomanometer, which should be used in clinical settings in which the paradox is anticipated but not elicited by palpation. With the cuff inflated above systolic pressure, Korotkoff sounds are meticulously sought over the brachial artery while the cuff is deflated at a rate of approximately 2 to 3 mm Hg per heart beat. This simple method permits identification of peak systolic pressure during *expiration*. When that pressure is identified and reconfirmed, the cuff is then deflated very slowly in order to identify *precisely* the pressure at which Korotkoff sounds become audible during expiration *and* inspiration. Pulsus paradoxus is present when the difference between the observed levels of peak systolic pressure at expiration and inspiration exceeds 10 mm Hg during quiet respiration.

Differential Pulsations and Selective Absence, Diminution, or Augmentation. Palpation of an artery can be used to grade a pulse from absent to augmented, permitting comparison with established norms for age, and comparison of right versus left and upper versus lower extremity pulses. A simple numerical system employs grades 0 to 4 +, with 0 as an absent pulse, 1 + as a present but diminished pulse, 2 + as an average normal pulse, 3 + as a moderately increased pulse, and 4 + as a markedly increased pulse. The information thus obtained is, in part, a variation on and an extension of the preceding sections that dealt with normal and abnormal wave forms of the arterial pulse.

The examination is more refined when a single digit rather than several fingertips is used to grade and compare arterial pulses. Sensitivity is not uniform in each digit, and the use of more than one finger may compromise the delicate control that is desirable when an artery is palpated. In most instances, I prefer to use the thumb for palpation as described above, because this apposable digit can be moved on its metacarpophalangeal hinge without bending the wrist, thus avoiding a position that decreases sensitivity in the fingertips. The thumb is convenient for simultaneous or sequential comparison of right and left arterial pulses (Fig. 3–20) and upper and lower extremity pulses (Fig. 3–23).

The circumstances under which one pulse is compared to another depends, in part, upon patient age. In infants and young children, the brachial and femoral pulses are routinely compared and graded. In adults, comparison and grading of arterial pulses include the carotids, brachials, radials, femorals, dorsalis pedis, and posterior tibial pulses.

The technique recommended for comparing contralateral pulses is shown in Figure 3–20. Brachial pulses are generally compared first as the examiner applies each thumb to the right and left antecubital fossae (Fig. 3–20A). In infants, the examiner must wait until the patient's arms are voluntarily quiet. Restraint more often than not provokes resistance, compromising rather than facilitating the examination. The brachial pulses can be compared during simultaneous palpation or with pressure applied in rapid succession while the thumb maintains contact with the overlying skin.

In adults, especially older adults, the most common cause of diminution or absence of a brachial pulse is atherosclerotic vascular disease. In younger patients, con-

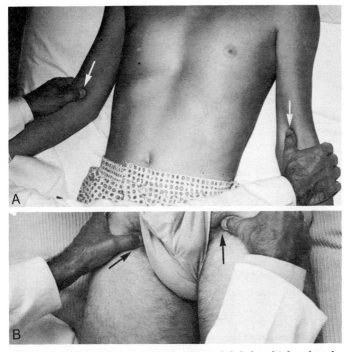

FIGURE 3–20. *A*, Comparison of right and left brachial pulses by simultaneous palpation with the thumbs *(arrows)*. *B*, Comparison of right and left femoral pulses by simultaneous palpation with the thumbs *(arrows)*.

genital malformations are the usual cause of differential right and left brachial pulsations. When coarctation of the aortic isthmus obstructs the orifice of the left subclavian artery, the *left* brachial pulse is diminished or absent, while the right brachial pulse is increased. When aortic stenosis is supravalvular, the right brachial pulse is greater than the left because of amplification of systolic pressure in the former. In adults (rarely in children), selective diminution of the *left* brachial pulse arouses suspicion of a subclavian steal. The suspicion is reinforced if palpation just above the left clavicle finds the ipsilateral subclavian pulse absent or diminished. Asym-

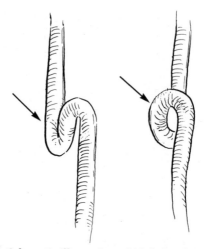

FIGURE 3–21. Schematic illustrations of kinked right carotid arteries.

metry of brachial pulses demands that blood pressure be determined in *both* arms irrespective of age.

The femoral arterial pulses are compared as the examiner applies the thumbs simultaneously to the right and left inguinal regions, as shown in Figure 3–20*B*. Comparative palpation of femoral pulses is not routinely performed in infants, children, or young adults but is obligatory in older patients in whom selective diminution occurs because of atherosclerotic obstruction.

In adults, especially older adults, the carotid arterial pulses routinely come under comparative assessment. Safety demands that comparison of right and left carotids be accomplished by *sequential* palpation, not by simultaneous compression (see Fig. 3–8). This qualification is necessary to minimize the risk of an undesirable decrease in cerebral blood flow if partially obstructed carotids are compressed simultaneously. Care should also be taken to avoid palpation in the vicinity of the carotid sinus, especially in elderly subjects.

Selective diminution of a carotid pulse is relatively common in older adults, but selective augmentation is unusual. An example of the latter is the kinked right carotid (Fig. 3–21). The kinked carotid is sometimes mistaken for a pulsating aneurysm, which it superficially resembles. When the carotid artery becomes too long for the distance it normally occupies, the vessel loops back sharply upon itself (Fig. 3–21), a change that occurs almost exclusively in the right carotid, and generally but not always beyond middle age, somewhat more frequently in women.[12]

Comparative palpation of the radial pulses is routine in adults. Best results are achieved by simultaneously applying the thumbs to the radial pulses while the patient's hands lie comfortably at the side with the palms supinated. Diminution or selective absence of a radial pulse, particularly in older adults, demands careful assessment of both radial and ulnar flow using Allen's test[13] (Fig. 3–22). Patency of the ulnar artery is assessed by occluding in sequence right and left radial arteries with the thumb while the patient briskly opens and closes the fist a dozen or so times (Fig. 3–22A and B). Selective arterial refilling is then judged by the rate of color return to the opened but not hyperextended palm, as pressure is maintained on the radial artery (Fig. 3–22D). Prompt return of normal color or transient reactive rubor of the palms and fingers indicates that the ulnar artery contributes normally to the circulation of the hand. Persistent pallor means ulnar occlusion. The test is then repeated while the right and left ulnar arteries are compressed to assess patency of the radials. The patient's fingers as well as the palm should be observed during sequential release of radial and ulnar arteries, because delayed flushing of an individual digit sometimes indicates local arterial obstruction.

The dorsalis pedis and posterior tibial arteries are routinely palpated in adults. Palpation with a fingertip is sometimes more convenient and sensitive than using the thumb. This is especially so when applying the index or middle finger to the posterior tibials. "Grabbing" the region of the posterior tibial artery with the tips of several fingers may initially help in identifying the pulse. Pulsations in the dorsalis pedis and posterior tibial arteries often vary from time to time in the same subject. Accordingly, diminution or absence during a single examination

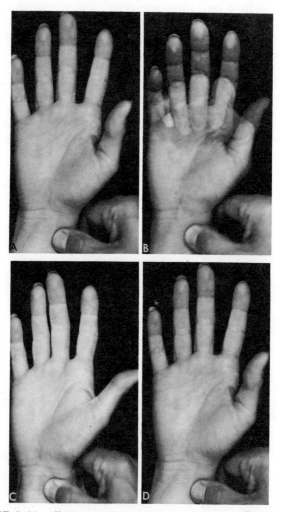

FIGURE 3–22. Allen's test illustrating assessment of ulnar arterial patency *(A)* by selective occlusion of the radial with the examiner's thumb. The patient briskly opens and closes the fist *(B)* to induce blanching *(C)*. While radial compression continues *(D)*, prompt return of color to the *opened* but *not hyperextended* palm and fingers is normal, indicating patency of the ulnar artery.

does not necessarily imply a persistent reduction in the pulse. A tablet of sublingual nitroglycerin often resolves doubt by rendering a temporarily absent dorsalis pedis or posterior tibial pulse readily palpable.

Let us now turn to comparison of *upper* versus *lower* extremity pulses (Fig. 3–23), a procedure that should be routine irrespective of age. Two methods have been advocated. Some examiners recommend comparison of femoral and *radial* arterial pulses, while others advocate

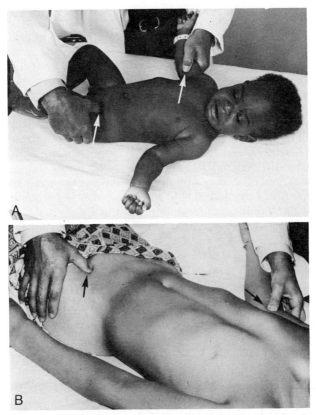

FIGURE 3–23. Comparison of brachial and femoral pulses by simultaneous palpation with the thumbs *(arrows)* in an infant *(A)* and a teenager *(B)*.

comparison of *brachial* and femoral arteries. The radial and femoral pulse waves are normally sensed as synchronous, so that *any* femoral delay is considered abnormal. Positioning the patient's wrist next to the groin brings the radial and femoral arteries into proximity, a technique believed to facilitate comparison. My preference is for simultaneous palpation of *brachial* and femoral arteries accomplished by placing a thumb on each (Fig. 3–23). In infants, especially newborns, palpation of the tiny radial pulse is impractical. When using the technique illustrated in Figure 3–23A, the examiner must wait for the baby voluntarily to relax its legs and arms. Restraint is counterproductive and may render a normal femoral pulse impalpable. When comparing the *brachial* and femoral pulses, the trivial normal delay in perceived arrival time of the femoral pulse (on the order of 15 milliseconds in adults, less in infants and children) is sensed as a norm against which even slight deviations are readily recognized. Furthermore, in all except a minority of patients with coarctation of the aorta, the femoral arterial pulses are *distinctly* reduced (Fig. 3–24), if not absent, so diagnostic differences between upper and lower extremity pulses are relatively apparent. In the occasional patient with mild coarctation, the femoral pulse is palpable, so that meticulous technique and timing are pivotal. In any event, what the examiner senses as femoral "delay" in coarctation of the aorta is not a delay in *arrival* of the femoral arterial pulse, but instead a delay in its rate of rise (damping) (Fig. 3–24).

In adults, especially older adults, a relative reduction in femoral compared to brachial arterial pulsations generally means atherosclerotic ileofemoral obstruction. In this setting, asymmetry of right versus left femoral pulse (see technique in Fig. 3–20B) is common.

Let us now turn to certain arterial pulses that are not routinely palpated but instead are examined only under certain circumstances that arouse suspicion. When peripheral arterial disease of the legs is suspected, popliteal arterial pulses should be palpated in addition to routine palpation of femorals, dorsalis pedis, and posterior tibials as described above. The techniques of popliteal arterial

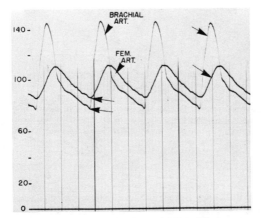

FIGURE 3–24. Brachial and femoral arterial pulses in coarctation of the aorta. The arrival times are virtually the same *(lower left arrows).* The difference perceived by the examiner during palpation reflects dissimilarity in the rates of rise (femoral slower than brachial) *(upper right arrows).*

palpation are shown in Figure 3–25. The more sensitive method (Fig. 3–25A) requires that the patient lie prone with knee flexed at less than a right angle and muscles relaxed by permitting the patient to rest the flexed leg against the shoulder of the examiner who sits or stands at the bedside or examining table. The midline of the popliteal fossa is palpated throughout its extent using the thumbs of both hands pressed firmly. An alternative method of palpating the popliteal artery is with the patient supine, the knee flexed, and the muscles relaxed while the examiner firmly applies the fingers of both hands to the midline of the popliteal fossa, as shown in Figure 3–25B).

In Chapter 2, brief comment was made on the skin of the foot in peripheral arterial occlusive disease. Diagnostic changes in color are elicited in the following manner. Examination begins with the patient supine. Each leg is then passively elevated, a maneuver that intensifies pallor in the ischemic limb, whereas the skin color of a limb with normal arterial circulation is not so affected. It is useful to elevate both legs simultaneously to induce or

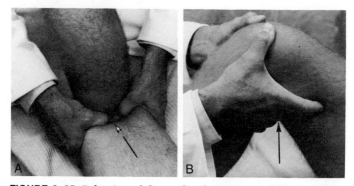

FIGURE 3–25. Palpation of the popliteal artery *(A)* while the patient is prone with knees flexed and muscles relaxed by resting the leg against the examiner's shoulder. The midline of the popliteal fossa is palpated using both thumbs *(arrow)* firmly pressed. *B,* Alternative method of palpating the popliteal artery (more convenient but less sensitive). With the patient supine, the knee is flexed and muscles relaxed while the fingers of both hands are firmly applied to the midline of the popliteal fossa *(arrow)*.

intensify the pallor. The patient should then change position promptly from supine to sitting with both legs lowered passively over the side of the bed or examining table. The rate of color return—which may be delayed for as long as 60 seconds—is then observed, and one foot is compared to the other. With return of color, continued dependency results in rubor (intensification of color) in the ischemic foot or in individual ischemic digits.

Digital pulsations (fingertips) are palpated under limited circumstances. Severe aortic regurgitation is an example. The patient's fingertips are gently but snugly gripped by the fingers of the examiner (Fig. 3–26). To be certain that the perceived pulsations are those of the patient and not of the clinician, the digital pulses can be timed by simultaneously palpating the ipsilateral radial artery while the patient's wrist is supported by the examiner's free hand (Fig. 3–26). The visual counterpart of increased digital pulsations in chronic severe aortic regurgitation is the Quincke pulse,[14] best elicited by transilluminating the fingertip with a small flashlight applied

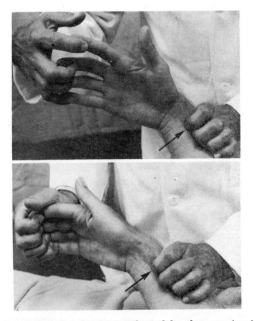

FIGURE 3–26. Digital pulsations palpated by the examiner's fingers snugly applied to the patient's fingertips. Although it is unlikely that the examiner will sense his or her own pulse, simultaneous palpation of the patient's radial pulse for timing purposes *(arrows)* provides confirmation.

to the skin opposite the nail in a darkened room. The examiner's free hand encloses the finger to provide a relatively focused field that highlights the phasic reddening and blanching of the nailbed with systole and diastole. Quincke wrote, "One observes a distinct . . . lightning-like and momentary accentuation of the reddening, so that the manner of the appearance and disappearance of the capillary pulse is objectively as characteristic a sign of aortic insufficiency as the exquisitely abrupt pulse to the palpating finger."[14]

Arterial Thrills and Murmurs. Arterial thrills and murmurs should be sought routinely over certain vessels, with the sites varying according to patient age. In normal children and young adults, an innocent supraclavicular systolic murmur can be sufficiently loud to produce a thrill. Auscultation should be performed while the patient sits and looks forward with the shoulders relaxed and the forearms and hands resting on the lap (Fig. 3–27A). The bell of the stethoscope is placed in the supraclavicular fossa over each subclavian artery. The shoulders are then hyperextended with the elbows brought sharply behind the back until the shoulder girdle muscles are taut (Fig. 3–27B). In response to this manuever, the innocent supraclavicular systolic murmur typically diminishes considerably or disappears altogether.

In adults, especially older adults, auscultation over carotid, subclavian, and femoral arteries is obligatory

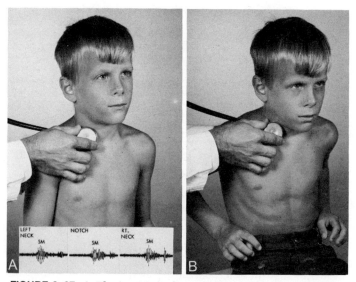

FIGURE 3–27. *A*, The inset is a phonocardiogram of a normal supraclavicular systolic murmur in the left and right neck and in the suprasternal notch. Auscultation begins as the patient sits with shoulders relaxed and forearms resting on the lap. *B*, When the shoulders are hyperextended by bringing the elbows well behind the back, the murmur typically diminishes or disappears.

even if palpation of these arteries is unrevealing. It is convenient to seek arterial murmurs at these sites at the time the pulses are initially palpated. Carotid and subclavian auscultation is achieved with the patient either supine or sitting and the patient's chin pointed straight ahead. The bell of the stethoscope is applied just firmly enough to achieve a skin seal over each internal carotid artery in its lower, middle, and upper thirds. A carotid arterial murmur is not necessarily louder on the side of a diminished pulse. In fact, the converse may be true. The right and left subclavian arteries are then examined by applying the stethoscope in the supraclavicular fossae. Femoral arterial auscultation requires that the patient lie supine while the bell of the stethoscope is applied sequentially over the right and left inguinal regions. Each femoral artery should be compared to the other, just as the carotids and subclavians are compared. A femoral arterial murmur is not necessarily louder on the side of a diminished pulse, a point that also applies to the carotid murmur, as already noted.

Nonroutine arterial auscultation is conducted at relatively unorthodox sites that are selected according to patient age and the examiner's clinical suspicion. When coarctation of the aortic isthmus is suspected, auscultation should be carried out in the posterior thorax over the site of the presumed coarctation. In infants, this observation is best made with the patient prone and the stethoscopic diaphragm firmly applied over the vertebral column between the scapulae. In older children and adults, auscultation for the same purpose can be accomplished with the patient sitting. The shoulders and thorax must be relaxed, and the diaphragm of the stethoscope is applied as just described. The murmur overlying the segment of coarctation can be systolic or continuous, depending upon the degree of aortic narrowing. The relatively high frequency of the murmur is the reason for using the stethoscopic diaphragm.

In older adults, auscultation is often appropriate over the abdominal aorta at its bifurcation, especially when palpation of the femoral arteries discloses ileofemoral atherosclerotic obstruction. In hypertensive patients, auscultation in the flanks over right and left kidneys may identify the soft, high-frequency systolic murmur that occasionally accompanies renal arterial obstruction (see Chapter 8).

Structural Properties. "We recognize the yielding nature of the arterial coats in healthy arteries. In degeneration of the coats, the arterial walls may be universally thickened or contain bead-like patches of induration as in atheroma, or the artery may have become a rigid tube, as in calcareous degeneration."[1] Structural abnormalities of systemic arteries are sometimes identified visually. The elongated tortuous brachial artery of Monckeberg's sclerosis is seen beneath the skin of the antecubital fossa (see Fig. 3–6) as each cardiac cycle imparts a distinctive snake-like movement to the tortuous vessel. Palpation, especially when the artery is "rolled" under the thumb, elicits the characteristic feel of a thickened, firm arterial wall as Mackenzie described. The radial arterial pulse and the dorsalis pedis pulse may also be seen as well as palpated, although only occasionally. Another case in point is the distinctive structural properties, both tactile and visual, of a kinked carotid artery (see Fig. 3–21) that may be mistaken for an aneurysm.

Conversely, true aneurysms are sometimes overlooked unless meticulously sought. An important example is an abdominal aortic aneurysm, especially in older adults with systemic hypertension (see Chapter 8). Pulsations of the normal abdominal aorta do not extend below the umbilicus, even in thin individuals with relatively flaccid abdominal walls. Accordingly, when abdominal pulsations extend below the umbilicus, an aortic aneurysm is the presumptive cause. Systolic murmurs in the vicinity of abdominal aortic aneurysms are more likely to originate from ileofemoral obstruction than within the aneurysm itself.

Femoral arterial aneurysms are, as a rule, readily identified when there is unilateral exaggeration of a femoral pulse, especially if that pulse is visible and the contralateral pulse is not. Small asymptomatic popliteal aneurysms, typically unilateral, are sometimes incidentally identified when the popliteal pulse is palpated as described earlier. The pulsation of an aneurysm in the popliteal fossa can be relatively apparent when the patient is examined prone with the knee flexed (see Fig. 3–25A). Less meticulous examination with the patient supine can miss an otherwise obvious popliteal aneurysm. Diagnosis depends upon assessment of the width of the pulsation when the fingers of both hands are firmly applied to the midline of the popliteal fossa.

REFERENCES

1. Mackenzie, J.: The Study of the Pulse, Arterial, Venous and Hepatic and of the Movements of the Heart. Edinburgh, Young J. Pentland, 1902.
2. Bedford, D. E.: The ancient art of feeling the pulse. Br. Heart J. 13:423, 1951.
3. Broadbent, W. H.: The Pulse. London, Cassell & Company, Limited, 1890.
4. Lewis, W. H.: The evolution of clinical sphygmomanometry. Bull. N.Y. Acad. Med. 17:871, 1941.
5. Korotkoff, N. S.: On methods of studying blood pressure. Bull. Imperial Military Acad. Med. (St. Petersburg) 11:365, 1905.
6. Segall, H. N.: How Korotkoff, the surgeon, discovered the auscultatory method of measuring arterial pressure. Ann. Intern. Med. 83:561, 1975.
7. Wood, F. C., and Wolferth, C. C.: Tolerance of certain cardiac patients for various recumbent positions (trepopnea). Am. J. Med. Sci. 193:354, 1937.
8. Wiggers, C. J.: The Pressure Pulses in the Cardiovascular System. London, Longmans, Green and Co., 1928.
9. Corrigan, D. J.: On permanent patency of the mouth of the aorta, or inadequacy of the aortic valve. Edinb. Med. Surg. J. 37:225, 1832.
10. Traube, L.: A case of pulsus bigeminus. Berl. Klin. Wochenschr. 9:185, 1872. Translated in Willius, F. A., and Keys, T. E. (eds.): Classics of Cardiology. Malabar, Florida, Robert E. Krieger Publishing Co., 1983.
11. Kussmaul, A.: Euber schweilige mediastinopericarditis und den paradoxen pulse. Klin. Wochenschr. 10:433, 1873.
12. Metz, H., Murray-Leslie, R. M., Bannister, R. G., Bull, J. W. D., and Marshall, J.: Kinking of the internal carotid artery in relation to cerebrovascular disease. Lancet 1:424, 1961.
13. Allen, E. V.: Thromboangiitis obliterans: Methods of diagnosis of chronic occlusive arterial lesions distal to the wrist with illustrative cases. Am. J. Med. Sci. 178:237, 1929.
14. Quincke, H.: Observations on capillary and venous pulse. Berl. Klin. Wochenschr. 5:357, 1868. Translated in Willius, F. A., and Keys, T. E. (eds.): Classics of Cardiology. Malabar, Florida, Robert E. Krieger Publishing Co., 1983.

THE VEINS—JUGULAR AND PERIPHERAL

This chapter deals first with the physical examination of the jugular veins—internal and external—as sources of anatomic, hemodynamic, and electrophysiologic information from the right atrium and right ventricle. The chapter then deals with the examination of veins of the extremities and thoracic inlet as reflections of primary, if not intrinsic, venous disease.

THE JUGULAR VEINS

In 1902, James Mackenzie[1] firmly established the jugular venous pulse as an important part of the cardiovascular physical examination.

> We come now to the study of a subject which gives us far more information of what is actually going on within the chambers of the heart. In the study of the venous pulse we have often the direct means of observing the effects of the systole and diastole of the right auricle, and of the systole and diastole of the right ventricle.

Despite this impetus, clinical analysis of the jugular pulse waned until Paul Wood, in the 1950's, reawakened interest, recalling that "precise analysis of the cervical venous pulse and measurement of the height of each individual wave with reference to the sternal angle is not only possible at the bedside but highly desirable."[2]

Information derived from examination of the jugular veins includes (1) wave form and pressure, (2) anatomic-physiologic inferences, and (3) arrhythmias and conduction defects. The technique of examination described below permits analysis of the jugular veins in most if not all patients, except infants whose short necks and inability to cooperate make examination of the jugular pulse impractical, although not impossible.

The External and Internal Jugular Veins. Examination of both of these veins is important, the external for estimates of mean right atrial pressure, the internal for wave form *and* pressure. The *internal* jugular vein, which is equipped with a bicuspid venous valve at the thoracic inlet, lies in the carotid sheath behind the sternocleidomastoid muscle, a clinically important anatomic relationship. The jugular bulb, a slight dilatation at the origin of the internal jugular (Fig. 4–1), lies in a hollow between the two clavicular insertions of the sternocleidomastoid muscle.

Phasic pressure imparted to the internal jugular vein accurately reflects the right atrial wave form. Accordingly, more information is derived from examination of the internal jugular pulse than from the external jugular vein, as Mackenzie observed: "The movements communicated by the heart to the blood in the veins are usually best observed in the internal jugular veins. The direct com-

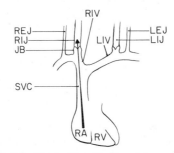

FIGURE 4–1. Sketch illustrating Mackenzie's contention that "the direct communication of the right internal jugular through the right innominate vein and superior vena cava in about a straight line renders it susceptible to the movements from the right heart."[1] REJ, RIJ = Right external and internal jugular; LEJ, LIJ = left external and internal jugular; RIV, LIV = right and left innominate veins; JB = jugular bulb; SVC = superior vena cava; RA = right atrium; RV = right ventricle.

munication of the right internal jugular through the right innominate and superior cava in about a straight line renders it susceptible to the movements of the right heart"[1] (Fig. 4–1). The *right* internal jugular vein is therefore more important than the left in the physical examination, because it provides a more accurate reflection of right atrial mechanical activity, and of right atrial and right ventricular pressure-volume relationships. Pulsations transmitted from the right atrium into the internal jugular vein are generated when the steady flow of systemic venous return becomes phasic upon reaching the right atrial chamber. The only significant difference between the wave forms of the right internal jugular vein and the right atrium is the impact of the carotid pulse on the former.

Normal Wave Form of the Internal Jugular Vein. Potain accurately described the wave form of the internal jugular vein in 1867,[3] and Mackenzie subsequently provided nomenclature that is used today with few or no significant modifications[1] (Fig. 4–2). Mackenzie designated the two crests as A and V, and went on to write:

> There are two rises in the auricular pressure curve—a large and a small one, with of course two falls. The first rise in pressure immediately precedes the rise in ventricular pressure. It can only be due to the systole of the auricle. Immediately after the auricle ceases to contract, there is a great fall *(x)* in the pressure due to the diastole of the auricle. The auriculo-ventricular valves being closed, the blood pouring into the auricles from the veins, the pressure gradually rises, producing the second small wave in the curve. This wave is terminated by the opening of the auriculo-ventricular valves at the beginning of the ventricular diastole . . . . When the pressure becomes lower in the ventricles than in the auricles the valves open and the contained blood passes through, reducing the auricular pressure, and causing the second fall, *y.* After this the pressure slowly rises by the accumulation of blood in both chambers, until it is suddenly increased by the next auricular systole.

These remarks require little elaboration. The A wave (Fig. 4–2A) reflects right atrial contraction and occurs just before the carotid arterial pulse and the first heart sound. The X descent (decline of the A wave) is initiated by right atrial relaxation and is reinforced as right ventricular contraction causes descent of the floor of the atrium. The

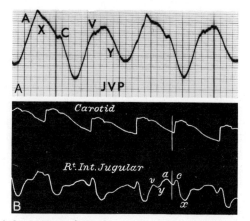

FIGURE 4–2. *A*, Normal jugular venous pulse (JVP) showing the A wave, the X descent interrupted by the C wave, and the V wave followed by the Y descent. *B*, James Mackenzie's "simultaneous tracings of the carotid pulse and the jugular pulse, showing the exact synchronism of the carotid wave (c) in the jugular pulse."[1] The designations of the crests and troughs of the jugular pulse are the same as those in tracing *(A)* above.

initial portion of the descent (atrial relaxation) is sometimes designated "X," while the remainder of the descent (during right ventricular contraction) is designated "X'." For practical bedside purposes, I use the standard designation "X" for the entire descent, while not ignoring the fact that the descent is due sequentially to right atrial diastole followed by descent of the floor of the right atrium during ventricular systole.

The X descent is often the most conspicuous feature of the normal jugular venous pulse and is interrupted by the C wave (Fig. 4–2) which, for all practical purposes, is the carotid impact itself. Mackenzie used the letter "C" to designate this movement, which he correctly ascribed to the carotid. A relatively small C wave is generated within the right atrium proper as right ventricular isovolumetric contraction displaces the tricuspid leaflets upward, but this wave is overshadowed in the jugular pulse by the much larger carotid pulsation with which it coincides.

The V wave (Fig. 4–2) was so designated by Mackenzie because its ascent begins during ventricular systole. The ascending limb of the V wave reflects passive filling of the right atrium as venous return continues in the face of a closed tricuspid valve. The Y descent represents sudden termination of the V wave as the right ventricle relaxes; the tricuspid valve then opens, and the right atrial pressure rapidly falls. The Y descent is normally less conspicuous than the X descent and the Y trough not as deep as the X trough (Fig. 4–2). The X descent is therefore the more obvious of the two declines.

Following the Y trough, right atrial and right ventricular pressures slowly rise in parallel (diastasis), especially when diastole is prolonged by a relatively slow heart rate. A slight rise preceding the next A wave is called the *h* wave, so designated by Hirschfelder in 1907.[4] The *h* wave is seldom seen in the normal jugular venous pulse except when the cardiac rate is slow.

Technique of Examination

Position of the Patient and Light Source. Proper examination of the jugular pulse requires that the patient lie supine on a bed or examining table that permits easily adjustable elevation of the trunk above the horizontal (Fig. 4–3). An electrically controlled bed adjustment is ideal. The patient's trunk should be positioned at an angle above the horizontal that corresponds to the maximum visible oscillations of the right internal jugular vein. I recommend beginning with a 30 to 40 degree elevation above the horizontal, then lowering or elevating the patient's trunk appropriately. If the central venous pressure is low, the trunk is lowered until venous pulsations become visible. If oscillations of the internal jugular are not seen within 15 degrees of the horizontal, gentle abdominal compression with the flat of the hand serves to increase venous return and transiently reveal the oscillations of the jugular pulse (see below, abdominojugular reflux). The higher the central venous pressure, the higher the required elevation of the patient's trunk above horizontal. If the jugular venous oscillations cannot

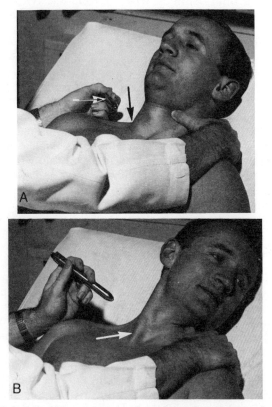

FIGURE 4–3. *A*, The patient's trunk is elevated 40 degrees above the horizontal. The head is adjusted to look forward or is rotated slightly to the right to relax the sternocleidomastoid muscle. The examiner's right thumb palpates the patient's left carotid for timing purposes, while a tangential light *(horizontal arrow)* shines across the right lower neck *(vertical arrow)* to highlight the crests and troughs of the jugular pulse. *B*, Rotating the head to the left tenses the sternocleido-mastoid muscle *(arrow)* and compresses or obliterates the jugular pulse. This position is to be avoided.

be seen with the patient sitting bolt upright, the legs should be dangled over the side of the bed or examining table, a maneuver that generally brings even very high jugular venous pulsations into view.

The patient's head should be adjusted (Fig. 4–3A) from a neutral position slightly upward or downward and to the right by gently moving the chin, but the head should not be tilted too far upward or turned sharply to the left, because these maneuvers tense the right sternocleidomastoid muscle (Fig. 4–3B) and compress or obliterate the underlying internal jugular pulse.

The light source is important. A small pocket flashlight usually suffices. The illumination should be directed tangentially across the area under examination (Fig. 4–3A) to highlight the shadows cast by the external jugular and the fluctuations of the internal jugular vein. It is convenient for the examiner to use the left hand to adjust the light source, leaving the right hand free to palpate the left carotid artery for timing purposes (Fig. 4–3A). The right hand can also be used to apply the stethoscope to the chest when the jugular pulse is timed with the heart sounds (see below).

The External Jugular Vein. The right external jugular vein may not be visible unless it is mechanically distended by digital compression at the root of the neck, as shown in Figure 4–4A. A distended right external jugular vein is recognized as a static, nonpulsatile column that is more apparent when it casts a shadow. Before using the crest of the external jugular as an estimate of mean right atrial pressure, two words of caution. First, venoconstriction occasionally obliterates the external jugular vein despite an elevation in mean right atrial pressure. Second, visible distention of the external jugular vein does not necessarily mean that the mean right atrial pressure is elevated. If the external jugular is not seen because of venoconstriction, examination of the pulsatile internal jugular vein prevents error (see below). If distention of the external jugular vein is not caused by an elevated mean right atrial pressure, the following simple maneuver makes this point. The distended vein is first emptied by applying digital pressure to its superior aspect

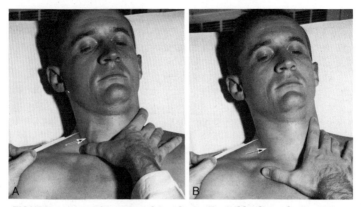

FIGURE 4–4. *A*, The external jugular vein visibly distends *(arrow)* as the vessel is compressed just above the clavicle. *B*, The distended vein disappears *(arrow)* when compression is released.

while blood is mechanically expressed from the vessel by running a thumb or finger downward along the vessel's course. The collapsed vein then lies between the two sites of digital compression. If selective release of the *inferior* site results in prompt filling from *below*, the cause is a high central venous pressure. As the vessel fills from below, the column of blood occasionally stops at a distinct bulge that represents a competent venous valve. If the external jugular does not fill from below, the maneuver can be repeated to identify filling from above. When the external jugular vein is once again mechanically emptied and the *superior* site of digital compression is released, distention of the vein indicates that filling is from above, which is generally of no clinical significance.

Except for these qualifications, the crest of the external jugular vein can be used as a convenient manometer for estimating mean right atrial pressure. When the patient's trunk is elevated 30 to 40 degrees above horizontal, the normal crest of the right external jugular vein is sometimes seen hovering just above the clavicle. Gentle digital compression at that site impedes flow from above and elevates the column (Fig. 4–4A); when compression is released, the crest of the column normally falls out of sight (Fig. 4–4B) or is seen just above the clavicle. In any event, the normal crest of the external jugular vein does not exceed 3 to 4 cm above the sternal angle. When the crest of a *distended* external jugular vein cannot be seen at 30 to 40 degrees above the horizontal, the patient's trunk should be elevated until the crest of the vein comes into view. The height of the crest is then measured in centimeters above the sternal angle, as shown in Figure 4–5.

The Internal Jugular Vein. Analysis of the wave form of the right internal jugular vein requires a reference for timing purposes, a recommendation made by Potain in 1867. "I studied them then in this relationship by combining palpation or auscultation of the precordial region with inspection of the cervical pulsations . . . ."[3] Mackenzie (1902) recommended using the carotid artery for timing purposes[1] (see Fig. 4–2B). The heart sounds provide still another reference. Examiner preference dictates whether the carotid arterial pulse or the heart sounds are

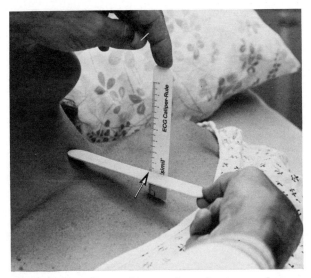

FIGURE 4–5. Use of a centimeter rule and a tongue depressor to measure the vertical distance *(arrow)* above the sternal angle of Louis.

used to time the jugular venous pulse. Both methods, properly applied, achieve the same end. I prefer the carotid because the physical examination does not have to be interrupted for auscultatory orientation, especially in patients with complex heart sounds and murmurs.

The examiner's right thumb palpates the patient's left carotid pulse, while the left hand is free to shine a tangential light across the undulations of the right internal jugular vein (see Fig. 4–3A). Cervical venous pulsations that are not synchronous with the carotid cannot be arterial and therefore must be venous. The A wave and the beginning of the X descent precede the carotid (C wave), which is immediately followed by the continuation of the X descent to its trough (see Fig. 4–2). The V wave begins just after the carotid pulse and is followed by the Y descent, after which an h wave is sometimes seen if diastole is sufficiently prolonged.

Timing of the jugular venous pulse with auscultation requires selection of a precordial site where the first and second heart sounds are easily heard. The examiner holds the stethoscope in place with the right hand while adjusting the light source with the left hand as described above. The first heart sound is just before the C wave (carotid pulse). The A wave and the beginning of the X descent precede the first heart sound. The remainder of the X descent (the portion of the normal jugular pulse that is more prominent during ventricular systole) proceeds beyond the first heart sound. The second heart sound immediately precedes the crest of the V wave, followed by the Y descent.

What the Eye Perceives. The normal jugular venous pulse is perceived as a series of gentle, undulating crests and troughs. The descents, especially the X descent, are usually more obvious to the eye than the crests. A relatively brisk X descent, for example, makes an otherwise subtle A wave apparent. The converse is the case with the carotid pulse, which is more obvious in its ascent than in its decline. Mackenzie recognized these points: "The sudden collapse of the tissues covering the vein is more striking than the protrusion, [whereas] . . . the carotid pulse is always abrupt and sudden in its protrusion of the covering tissues, and gradual in its shrinking."[1]

The Effects of Respiration. "When the steady stream of venous blood approaches the heart, it is subjected to the intermittent influences of the respiratory and cardiac actions."[1] The jugular venous pulse often becomes more obvious during inspiration, and a low normal jugular pulse is sometimes evident *only* during inspiration. This is so chiefly because the descents, especially the X descent, become brisker during inspiration and therefore more apparent to the eye. During the inspiratory fall in intrathoracic pressure, *mean* right atrial and jugular venous pressures decline despite an increased venous return. The increase in venous return, however, serves to augment right atrial contractile force and to preserve or increase the crest of the A wave, setting the stage for accentuation of the first portion of the X descent as the right atrium relaxes after a more vigorous contraction. In addition, the inspiratory augmentation in right ventricular volume and contractile force results in an increase in systolic descent of the floor of the right atrium and accordingly in an increase of the portion of the X descent that follows the C wave. The Y descent is brisker during inspiration (although not as impressively so as the X descent) because tricuspid flow during the rapid filling phase is reinforced by the inspiratory fall in right ventricular diastolic pressure. A distinction should be made between the *normal* cervical venous response to inspiration, namely, a jugular pulse that is more readily perceived but at a lower mean pressure, and an *abnormal* response to inspiration, namely, a *rise* in right atrial mean and jugular venous pressures (Kussmaul's sign, see below).

The Jugular Venous Pulse Versus the Carotid Pulse. This difference, mentioned earlier, requires elaboration. "The pulse in the internal jugular vein is often mistaken by most experienced observers for 'beating of the carotids.' "[1] The carotid pulse has a single rise and fall, whereas the jugular pulse has two crests and two troughs. The *rise* of the carotid is brisker (more visible) than its descent, whereas the jugular venous descents are more obvious than their crests. Inspiration diminishes the carotid pulse but makes the jugular pulse more obvious. Abdominal compression (see below) has no effect on the carotid but transiently improves visibility of the jugular pulse. The carotid artery is normally palpable, whereas the jugular pulse is not. Sitting improves visibility of the carotid pulse, while the jugular venous pulse drops from sight. Gentle digital compression just above the clavicle obliterates the internal jugular venous pulse but not the carotid, as Potain recognized. "A light pressure, suitably applied to the lower portion of the neck can impede them or suppress them entirely, while the pulsations of the carotid persist with all of their intensity."[3]

The Hepatic Pulse. The right atrial pulse is transmitted into the internal jugular vein via the superior vena cava (see Fig. 4–1), while the liver pulse (Figs. 4–6 and 4–7) is transmitted via the inferior vena cava. "The relationship between the liver pulse and the jugular pulse is a very intimate one. . . . In certain cases, waves of blood are sent back into the inferior vena cava, and these waves distend the liver, and give rise to a pulsatile swelling of the organ. When there is both a venous and a liver pulse present they are always of the same character, and one can demonstrate the changes that take place by the liver pulse as well as by the venous pulse"[1] (Figs. 4–6 and 4–7).

The hepatic pulse is detected by palpation rather than by inspection, while the converse is true for the jugular

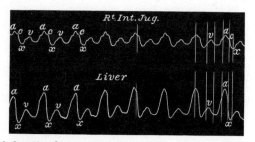

FIGURE 4–6. "Simultaneous tracings of the jugular and liver pulses" (Mackenzie[1]). The major wave forms are similar except for absence of the carotid (c) wave in the hepatic pulse.

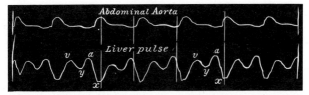

FIGURE 4–7. "Simultaneous tracings of the abdominal aorta and of the . . . liver pulse" (Mackenzie[1]). The wave form of the liver pulse is not altered by the aorta.

pulse. The examiner should place the palm of the right hand upon the patient's right upper quadrant below the liver edge. Care should be taken to avoid bending the wrist, which decreases sensitivity in the fingertips as they establish contact with the liver edge. A normal, gentle liver pulse is sometimes detectable in thin individuals with flaccid abdominal walls. When the liver is palpable during normal respiration, the patient is instructed to breathe as quietly as possible, or preferably to hold the breath briefly in a comfortable respiratory midposition. If the liver is not readily palpable, the patient is asked to take a moderately deep breath and hold it just long enough to permit accurate palpation of the descended liver edge.

Assessment of Central Venous Pressure. The term "jugular venous distention" is imprecise and is best avoided when describing the venous pulse or pressure. The examiner should focus first on the nonpulsatile *external* jugular vein (see Fig. 4–4) and then on the height of the A and V crests of the *internal* jugular vein as discussed here. Before estimating the central venous pressure, the patient's trunk should be adjusted above the horizontal to an angle that coincides with the maximal excursions of the right internal jugular vein. The head is then positioned to minimize compression by the sternocleidomastoid muscle (see Fig. 4–3).

The reference level against which venous pressure is measured is the sternal angle of Louis (Pierre Charles Alexandre Louis, 1787–1872), as Paul Wood recommended.[2] The angle of Louis is a well-defined ridge at the junction of the sternum and the manubrium (Fig. 4–8). This reference point was originally chosen because of the assumption that a relatively constant relationship existed between the sternal angle and the center of the right atrium whether the patient was supine, sitting, or reclining at some angle in between. Although the assumption should not be taken literally, use of the sternal angle as the zero reference is simple and practical and provides a reproducible and readily identified standard for bedside appraisal of venous pressure.

Three venous beds are available for estimation of pressure—the external jugular vein (see above), the internal jugular vein, and veins on the dorsa of the hands (see "The Upper Extremities").

The *right internal* jugular vein permits assessment of the heights of the A and V crests, just as the nonpulsatile *external* jugular permits an approximation of mean right atrial pressure (see Fig. 4–5). With the patient's trunk elevated 30 to 40 degrees above the horizontal, normal A and V waves undulate just above the clavicle, with the A wave slightly dominant (see Fig. 4–2). When related to the sternal angle as a reference, the crests of the normal A and V waves do not exceed 3 to 4 cm above the angle of Louis when the patient's trunk is 40 degrees above the horizontal.

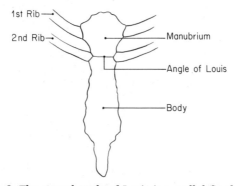

FIGURE 4–8. The sternal angle of Louis is a well-defined transverse ridge or junction between the manubrium above and the body of the sternum below.

In judging the jugular venous pressure, the response to abdominal compression can be useful. The term "hepatojugular reflux" was coined by Rondot in 1898,[6] although observations on the response of the cervical veins to abdominal compression were published in England a few years earlier.[7] Right upper quadrant pressure generally provokes the most pronounced response, but neither enlargement nor compression of the liver is required to elicit the response. Accordingly, simplicity recommends the alternative term "abdominal compression" rather than either "hepatojugular reflux" or "abdominojugular reflux."

The technique of applying abdominal pressure is important. The patient is instructed to relax and breathe as quietly as possible. The examiner gently applies the palm of the right hand to the center of the patient's abdomen (periumbilical), as illustrated in Figure 4–9. Relaxation of the abdomen requires that the examiner's hand be comfortably warm and that the initial contact be gentle. When the patient is breathing quietly and accustomed to the presence of the examiner's hand, compression begins—gently, gradually, progressively—and continues until the desired rise in jugular venous pressure is observed while the examiner scrutinizes the cervical veins with a flashlight held in the left hand. Abdominal compression is maintained for at least 30 seconds (at most 1 minute)

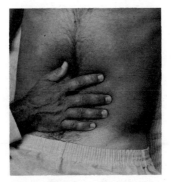

FIGURE 4–9. The abdominojugular reflux is performed with the palm of the hand gently but firmly applied to the center of the abdomen.

while the external and internal jugular veins are observed. This method is designed to minimize the likelihood of inadvertent straining (the Valsalva maneuver) or of increased respiratory excursions which interfere with, if not cancel, the desired response. "Warning" the patient often causes anxious anticipation and is best avoided. Rapid pressure provokes reflex abdominal tension. Pressure applied to the right upper quadrant in the presence of congestive hepatomegaly may be painful, while central abdominal pressure, as illustrated in Figure 4–9, avoids the tender liver.

The normal response to the augmented venous return caused by abdominal compression is a transient increase in prominence of the external jugular vein and of the crests and troughs of the internal jugular vein. This initial increase is followed *after a few beats* by a fall to control levels as abdominal compression continues. If the initial rise in jugular venous pressure is *not* followed promptly by a fall but instead is maintained during the entire 30 seconds to 1 minute of abdominal compression, right ventricular failure is the most common cause. An abnormally sustained response to abdominal compression also occurs with constrictive pericarditis and tricuspid stenosis. In the presence of emphysema or bronchospastic pulmonary disease, abdominal compression may result in an abnormal rise in jugular venous pressure in the absence of right ventricular failure, presumably because a sudden, disproportionate increase in intrathoracic pressure impedes venous return.

Anatomic-Hemodynamic Inferences

Observations of abnormal wave forms of the right internal jugular vein permit relatively precise anatomic and hemodynamic inferences. The A wave, the X descent, the V wave, the Y descent, and occasionally the h wave all come under scrutiny.

The A Wave. A giant A wave " . . . leaps to the eye, towering above and dwarfing the other waves of the venous pulse . . . ."[2] Such a dramatic event has its reasons, as the following story illustrates.

One afternoon when I was seeing outpatients with Dr. Wood at the National Heart Hospital, he stood beside an examining table and looked intently at the neck of a young woman. Wood's comments went something like this: "The pulsation in the neck is extraordinarily large. Even from this distance, I can see amplification during inspiration, implying that the pulse is venous. Its regularity implies sinus rhythm. Assuming that this is so, the pulse must be a giant A wave caused by powerful right atrial contraction that meets a resistance. The resistance can only be at the tricuspid orifice (tricuspid stenosis) or within a thick-walled hypertrophied right ventricle (severe pulmonic stenosis or hypertension with intact ventricular septum)." Wood then leaned forward and palpated the left sternal edge. He remarked, "There is no right ventricular impulse, no thrill of pulmonic stenosis. Nor can I feel the pulmonic component of the second heart sound. The A wave, therefore, cannot be due to pulmonic stenosis or pulmonary hypertension, so this young woman must have tricuspid stenosis." And she did!

Neither a word nor an inference need be changed. Giant A waves are generated when a forceful right atrium contracts against an appreciable resistance at one of two levels—an obstructed tricuspid orifice or within the cavity of the thick-walled hypertensive right ventricle of severe pulmonic stenosis or pulmonary hypertension with intact ventricular septum. Wood called the giant A wave the "venous Corrigan,"[2] indicating that he, like Dominic Corrigan, was referring to the *visual* image created by the dramatic pulse in the neck (see Chapter 3).

In dealing with increased A waves, all gradations exist from mild at one end of the spectrum to giant at the other (Fig. 4–10). At the mild end of the spectrum, the A wave is likely to be seen as abrupt and flicking before its crest is conspicuously elevated. Inspiration or abdominal compression reinforces this impression by transiently increasing the venous return and augmenting the X descent.

In sinus rhythm, the A wave regularly precedes the carotid pulse. If A waves are present but do not conform

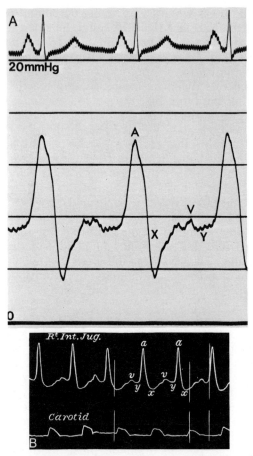

FIGURE 4–10. *A,* Giant A wave in a woman with severe rheumatic tricuspid stenosis. *B,* "When the auricular wave is large and stands out clear and distinct from other elements, it is evidence of a powerful right auricle" (Mackenzie[1]). Compare with *A.*

to this sequential relationship to the carotid, or if A waves are absent altogether, disturbances in rhythm or conduction are the cause (see below).

The X Descent. The X descent can be either more or less conspicuous than normal. An increase in the initial portion of the X descent represents enhanced right atrial relaxation following augmented contraction that might be due to the normal inspiratory increase in venous return, or to the increased force of right atrial contraction that generates the giant A wave described above. An increase in the briskness of the second (later) portion of the X descent (descent of the floor of the right atrium) occurs in response to augmented right ventricular contraction. Augmentation in right ventricular contractile force can be due to an increase in afterload or preload. An important variation on this theme is the conspicuous X descent

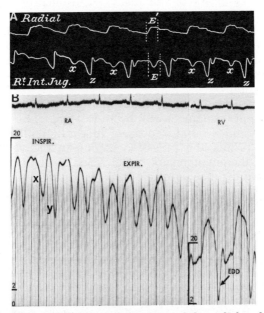

FIGURE 4–11. *A,* "Simultaneous tracings of the radial and jugular pulses, showing a great depression occurring during the ventricular diastole. From a case of chronic mediastinitis" (Mackenzie[1]). "E" is the period of "ejection" (ventricular systole). "Z" is the trough of the brisk "y" descent. *B,* The right atrial (RA) pulse in constrictive pericarditis showing a conspicuous "x" descent and an even brisker and deeper "y" descent, in addition to Kussmaul's sign—inspiratory increase in the right atrial pressure pulse. The right ventricular (RV) tracing shows an early diastolic dip (EDD, *arrow*) that coincides with the "y" descent.

of constrictive pericarditis due chiefly, if not exclusively, to enhanced descent of the floor of the right atrium during right ventricular systole (Fig. 4–11).

Blunting of the X descent can also be diagnostically important. In the normal heart, the X descent is brisker and deeper than the Y descent, as mentioned earlier and as shown in Figure 4–2. Blunting of the X trough is an early sign of tricuspid regurgitation, which cancels the latter part of the X descent that coincides with right ventricular systole (Fig. 4–12).

The V Wave and the Y Descent. "One constantly finds clinical evidence of the ready occurrence of tricuspid incompetence in the study of the venous pulse."[1] In pure tricuspid regurgitation in sinus rhythm, the ascent of the V wave is earlier in systole, its crest is higher, and the Y descent is brisk (Fig. 4–12). The tall V wave is sometimes called a "systolic venous wave," which is an appropriate designation.

The jugular pulse of tricuspid regurgitation in atrial fibrillation is characterized by an isolated tall, even giant V wave and a rapid Y descent (diastolic collapse) (Fig. 4–13). "When the pulsation is due to the ventricular systole, the engorgement of the veins is usually so great, the arterial pulse so small, and the cardiac mischief so evident, that the recognition of the venous pulse is comparatively easy."[1]

In the presence of tricuspid regurgitation with a tall V

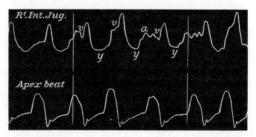

FIGURE 4–12. "Simultaneous tracings of the jugular pulse and of the apex beat" in a patient "during an attack of heart failure" (from Mackenzie[1]). Tricuspid regurgitation had caused blunting of the X descent and an increase in the height of the v wave.

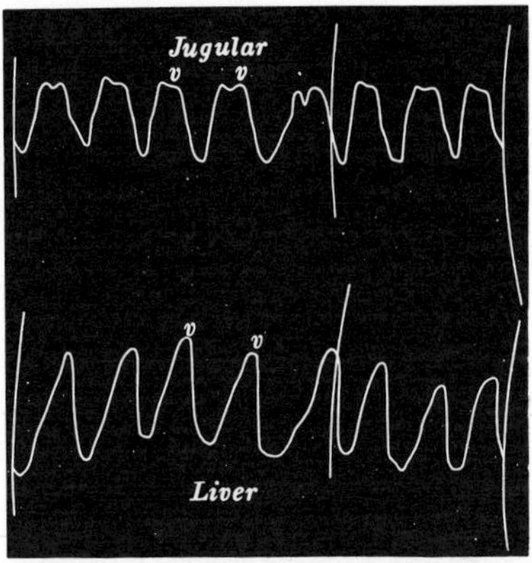

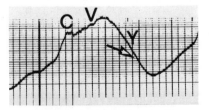

FIGURE 4–13. In this figure, "the venous and liver pulses of the ventricular type are given" (Mackenzie[1]). The tracings show the large v waves and brisk, if not collapsing, y descents of tricuspid regurgitation in the jugular venous pulse and in the liver pulse.

wave, the valve of the internal jugular vein becomes incompetent. Disproportionate systolic filling of the *right* internal jugular vein—which is in direct line with the right atrium, right innominate vein and superior vena cava (see Fig. 4–1)—results in a right-to-left "head bob," best seen when the examiner observes the patient frontally.

A tall V wave with a *rapid* fall of the Y descent indicates that the tricuspid orifice is unobstructed. Conversely, a tall V wave with an inappropriately *slow* Y descent is a feature of obstruction at the tricuspid orifice, usually

FIGURE 4–14. The jugular venous pulse in tricuspid stenosis with atrial fibrillation. The ascent of the V wave is not increased (trivial tricuspid regurgitation). Despite a tall V crest, the Y descent *(arrow)* is slow.

rheumatic tricuspid stenosis with atrial fibrillation (Fig. 4–14). The rate of rise of the *ascending* limb of the V wave is not increased (Fig. 4–14), because the right atrium fills chiefly, if not exclusively, from the venae cavae, indicating that coexisting tricuspid regurgitation is mild or absent. The Y descent is slow despite the tall V crest because the stenotic tricuspid orifice puts an effective brake on the rate of right ventricular filling despite high right atrial pressure.

A modest increase in V wave *without* tricuspid regurgitation is a subtle, minor, but interesting sign of a large atrial septal defect. The crests of the A and V waves in the jugular pulse become equal in height when a nonrestrictive atrial septal defect permits transmission of the *left* atrial wave form into the *right* atrium and internal jugular vein (Fig. 4–15).

Amplification of A and V Waves. The most common cause of an increase in A *and* V waves is right ventricular failure. Both crests are increased, but the A wave remains dominant as long as the tricuspid valve is relatively

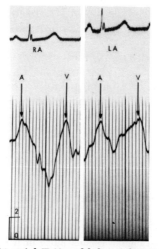

FIGURE 4–15. Right atrial (RA) and left atrial (LA) pressure pulses in a nonrestrictive ostium secundum atrial septal defect. The A and V waves are equal in height and resemble a left atrial pressure pulse.

competent. A subtle but sometimes useful point is the modification of the later part of the X descent which becomes less brisk and more shallow because of diminished right ventricular systolic contribution to its descent (depressed right ventricular contractility). Rarely, right ventricular failure is associated with tall A and V waves that "alternate"—right atrial pulsus alternans (Fig. 4–16).

Pulmonary hypertensive right ventricular failure with tricuspid regurgitation expresses itself in the jugular venous pulse as an increase in A and V waves with diminished X descent and a prominent if not collapsing Y trough. Pulmonary hypertension generates the large A wave, and tricuspid regurgitation blunts the X descent and increases the V crest and Y descent.

The A and V waves may be high and equal, yet their pulsations inconspicuous as in chronic constrictive pericarditis (see Fig. 4–11). This type of jugular pulse is recognized chiefly by the brisk X and Y descents (see Fig. 4–11), often best seen with the patient sitting bolt upright. The most consistent feature is the rapid Y descent to which the term "diastolic collapse" was originally applied by Friedreich in 1864.[8] Very high but relatively nonpulsatile A and V crests punctuated by rapid X and

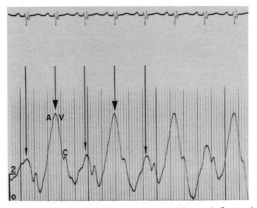

FIGURE 4–16. Right atrial alternans *(arrows)* in an infant with severe pulmonic valve stenosis and right ventricular failure. Tachycardia has caused the A and V waves to summate.

Y descents impart a W-shaped pattern to the jugular pulse of chronic constrictive pericarditis. Inspiration increases the rate of fall of X and Y descents but may not significantly affect the A and V crests, except as expressed in Kussmaul's sign.[9] When the crests of the A and V waves are visible (the patient may have to sit or stand), inspiratory augmentation in venous return results in a distinct, abnormal *increase* in mean right atrial pressure and in A and V crests (see Fig. 4–11B) because the constricted right ventricle cannot accept the inspiratory increase in volume without an increase in its filling pressure. Kussmaul's sign is still applied to an abnormal inspiratory increase in internal jugular venous pressure.

The "h" Wave. The *h* wave is briefly mentioned as a matter of completion. In 1907, Alexander G. Gibson wrote, "In the course of a study of jugular pulses in normal persons, I have noticed that in those whose pulse rate is slower than the average a wave between the 'v' wave and 'a' wave is often to be seen."[10] The *h* wave also becomes visible when diastasis occurs at a high level of right atrial pressure in the presence of a relatively slow heart rate. This is so because flow from a high-pressure right atrium into a right ventricle with impaired diastolic distensibility results in a prominent Y trough followed by a steep ascent to a plateau, the onset of which is sometimes seen as the *h* wave.

The Hepatic Pulse. The relative ease and clarity with which *jugular* venous pulsations are accessible cast the hepatic pulse into a secondary role. Nevertheless, "in many cases the changes in volume of the liver offer a most constructive indication of the condition of the circulation."[1] Palpation of the liver is a routine part of the cardiac physical examination that can be extended to identify a liver pulse as described earlier. Search for a liver pulse is relevant when examination of the jugular pulse predicts transmission of an abnormal right atrial wave form into the liver via the inferior vena cava. The examiner's fingertips perceive movements that coincide with the wave form of the jugular pulse (see Figs. 4–6 and 4–7). The timing of hepatic pulsations is easier when there is selective amplification of either the presystolic or the systolic liver pulse. Mackenzie remarked, "In tricuspid stenosis, when the auricle at first hypertrophies, the waves sent back by the auricle are of sufficient strength to cause a marked pulsation in the liver."[1] The liver pulse is most dramatic in severe tricuspid regurgitation with hepatomegaly because the right ventricle ejects across the incompetent tricuspid valve into the inferior vena cava and directly into the hepatic bed (see Fig. 4–13). In this setting, systolic movement of the liver may not only impart visible motion to the right upper quadrant of the abdomen, but also to the right lower thorax. Severe tricuspid regurgitation with hepatomegaly results in systolic *expansion* of the liver identified by placing the palpating right hand upon the right upper quadrant while the left hand is applied directly posterior at the margin of the lower ribs.

Electrophysiologic Inferences—Arrhythmias and Conduction Defects

"I had been endeavoring to discriminate between the different forms of irregular heart action and it occurred to me to employ the jugular pulse as an aid. By this means I was able to separate the great majority of irregularities into definite groups, according to the mechanism of their production . . . ."[1]

H. J. L. Marriott's advice in diagnosing cardiac arrhythmias from the electrocardiogram, "cherchez le P," can be applied in principle to the jugular venous pulse—"cherchez le A." Electrocardiographic analysis of complex arrhythmias requires identification of atrial and ventricular activity and their relationship to each other. The A and V waves of the jugular venous pulse provide the clinician with an analogous opportunity. Occasionally, the A wave is better seen in the jugular pulse than the P wave in the electrocardiogram. Arrhythmias that can be recognized in the jugular venous pulse are shown in Table 4–1.

The slow cardiac rate and regular rhythm of *sinus bradycardia* are identified by the normal, regular sequence of A wave preceding V wave. However, 2:1 sino-

TABLE 4–1. Arrhythmias Recognized in the Jugular Pulse

Sinus bradycardia
Sinus arrhythmia
Ectopic or premature beats (atrial, junctional, ventricular)
Ectopic tachycardias or ectopic rhythms (atrial, junctional, ventricular)
Loss of co-ordinated atrial activity (atrial fibrillation)

atrial exit block is indistinguishable from sinus bradycardia in the jugular pulse, as it is in the electrocardiogram. *Sinus arrhythmia* is recognized by confirming that the rate accelerations occur only during inspiration and are abolished when the breath is held in the respiratory midposition, while the A-C-V sequence in the jugular pulse remains normal and unchanged (Fig. 4–17). *Premature atrial beats* are recognized by cycles that begin early but preserve the normal sequence of A wave, carotid pulse, and V wave. The changes in cycle length prompted by premature atrial beats are distinguished from the changes in cycle length of sinus arrhythmia because the latter, not the former, are abolished during held respiration. In older subjects, premature atrial beats may be accompanied by pauses owing to prolonged sinus reset times. These pauses should not be mistaken for the true compensatory pauses that follow premature ventricular beats. Error is avoided by observing in the jugular pulse of atrial premature beats the normal relationship between A wave and carotid pulse as described above.

The term *cannon wave* refers to amplification of the A wave when right atrial contraction coincides with closure of the tricuspid valve. In *junctional* or *ventricular* pre-

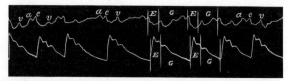

FIGURE 4–17. "Simultaneous tracings of the jugular and radial pulses, showing agreement in rhythm of the right auricle and ventricle (waves a and v), with the radial pulse, in the youthful form of irregularity." In this tracing, Mackenzie illustrated sinus arrhythmia.[1] "E" is the period of ejection (ventricular systole).

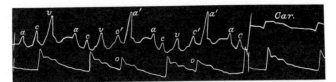

FIGURE 4–18. "Simultaneous tracings of the jugular and radial pulse. The auricular wave following a' occurs earlier, as if to take on the ventricular rhythm."[1] Mackenzie's tracings illustrate cannon A waves (a') occurring with premature ventricular beats ("o") as identified in the radial pulse.

mature beats (Fig. 4–18), cannon waves are the rule because right atrial systole finds the tricuspid valve closed by the premature ventricular contraction. Accordingly, cannon waves distinguish ventricular premature beats with compensatory pauses from atrial premature beats with prolonged sinus reset times as noted above. Cannon waves occur with junctional premature beats whether or not the premature beats are accompanied by retrograde atrial activation (Fig. 4–19). In either case, atrial activation coincides with ventricular systole, generating cannon A waves.

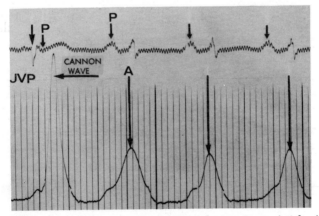

FIGURE 4–19. Cannon A wave *(horizontal arrow)* associated with retrograde atrial activation (first P wave) in a patient with a junctional premature beat *(first upper vertical arrow).*

Recognition of *ectopic tachycardias* is, in part, an extension of the discussion of ectopic beats. For example, the continuous beat-to-beat cannon A waves in *junctional tachycardia* (Fig. 4–20) are merely sustained examples of the mechanism generating the intermittent cannon waves of junctional premature beats (see Fig. 4–19). Sustained junctional rhythm with rates above 100 beats per minute is called junctional tachycardia, and below 100 beats per minute junctional rhythm. In *paroxysmal supraventricular tachycardia* (generally re-entrant), a discernible A wave precedes each carotid pulse, provided that the rate is not excessive. With rates above 160 beats per minute, A and V waves merge (blend) into a single venous crest followed by a single descent. Mackenzie's description is relevant (Fig. 4–21): "With still greater increase of the pulse rate, the ventricular wave *v* becomes shortened even to such an extent that its rise is blended into that of the auricular wave, so that only one true venous pulse wave is recognized."[1] These summated A and V crests resemble the beat-to-beat cannon waves of junctional tachycardia (Fig. 4–20), the distinction lying chiefly in the difference in rates. Paroxysmal supraventricular

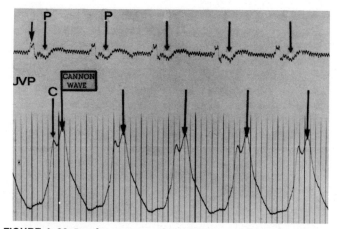

FIGURE 4–20. Jugular venous pulse (JVP) in a patient with junctional rhythm *(first upper vertical arrow)*, 1:1 retrograde atrial activation (P waves), and regular, sustained cannon waves. C = Carotid.

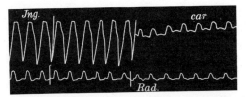

FIGURE 4–21. "Simultaneous tracings of the pulsation in the jugular bulb and in the radial, and of the carotid and radial pulses, during an attack of paroxysmal tachycardia, taken eighteen hours from the beginning of the attack."[1] Mackenzie's illustration shows regular cannon waves in the jugular pulse (Jng.) [sic] coinciding with each ventricular systole in the radial (Rad.) pulse. The rate is very rapid. car = Carotid.

tachycardia is usually associated with rates of 160 to 250 beats per minute, whereas in junctional tachycardia, the rates are slower, generally not much above 100 beats per minute.

Ventricular tachycardia with 1:1 retrograde atrial activation results in beat-to-beat cannon waves indistinguishable from those of junctional tachycardia. More commonly, however, ventricular tachycardia produces a fundamentally different jugular venous pulse, because atrial activity is *independent* of ventricular activity (atrioventricular dissociation). Accordingly, ventricular tachycardia is recognized in the jugular pulse by a regular rhythm and rapid rate as judged by palpation of the carotid, accompanied by independent A waves at a rate slower than that in the carotid. Importantly, and often distinctively, fortuitous atrial contraction against a closed tricuspid valve results in intermittent amplification of right atrial beats—cannon A waves. Accordingly, regular tachycardia occurring with slower independent A waves and intermittent cannon waves is characteristic of ventricular tachycardia. This observation is useful in distinguishing ventricular tachycardia from supraventricular tachycardia with aberrant ventricular conduction when P waves cannot confidently be identified in the electrocardiogram.

Atrial flutter is typically represented by co-ordinated atrial activity at rates of about 300 beats per minute, and a regular ventricular response at 150 beats per minute (2:1 atrioventricular block). The ease with which flutter waves can be seen in the jugular venous pulse (Fig. 4–22) depends chiefly upon the condition of the right atrium prior to the onset of atrial flutter. If sinus rhythm with large A waves is replaced by atrial flutter, the flutter waves are likely to be relatively conspicuous, as shown in Figure 4–22. Carotid sinus massage transiently slows the ventricular response, facilitating detection of flutter waves in the jugular pulse. Similarly, when flutter occurs with a higher degree AV block (generally 4:1), flutter waves are easier to identify in the jugular pulse because of the relatively long diastoles. In addition, the flutter waves may amplify in bursts when the right atrium flutters against a closed tricuspid valve (Fig. 4–22).

Atrial fibrillation is recognized in the jugular venous pulse by absence of co-ordinated atrial activity, a sine qua non for the diagnosis. Loss of A waves in the presence of an irregular rhythm as identified in the carotid pulse is typical and distinguishes the irregular rhythm of atrial fibrillation from the irregular rhythm of multiple premature atrial or ventricular beats in which A waves are present and often distinctive, as described earlier. Because of the absence of right atrial contraction and relaxation in atrial fibrillation, the initial portion of the X

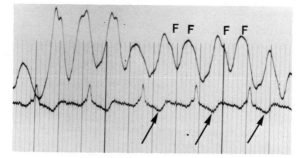

FIGURE 4–22. Prominent flutter waves (F) amplifying in bursts in the jugular venous pulse of a young woman with rheumatic mitral stenosis. In the electrocardiogram, arrows point to flutter waves.

**TABLE 4–2. Conduction Defects Recognized
in the Jugular Pulse**

PR interval prolongation
Wenckebach periods
Second-degree heart block
Complete atrioventricular block

descent is missing, so the X trough is relatively inconspicuous.

Conduction defects recognized in the jugular pulse are listed in Table 4–2. The PR *interval* can be estimated by the interval between the A wave and carotid pulse. The practiced eye comes to recognize normal, prolonged or short AC (and therefore PR) intervals. The cause of an increase in AC (or PR) interval is prolongation of atrioventricular conduction. Complete *left bundle branch block* also prolongs the AC interval, albeit slightly, by delaying left ventricular activation. A corollary of AC prolongation applies to recognition of *Wenckebach periodicity* that is characterized in the jugular pulse by gradual lengthening of sequential AC intervals, ending with an A wave that is not followed by a carotid pulse (nonconducted beat). Wenckebach periods (Mobitz I) differ from Mobitz II atrioventricular block, which is recognized in the jugular pulse by AC intervals that do not vary but are suddenly interrupted by isolated A waves that are not followed by a carotid pulse (nonconducted beat). *Two-to-one atrioventricular block* is recognized by two A waves for every one carotid pulse (Fig. 4–23). The blocked, isolated A waves differ somewhat from those that immediately precede a carotid pulse; their X descent is blunted because only its initial portion (right atrial

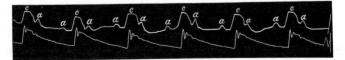

FIGURE 4–23. "Tracings of the pulsation in the neck due to a wave, *a*, in the jugular vein and the carotid pulse, *c*, taken at the same time as the radial. There are two auricular waves, *a*, to one carotid pulse."[1] Mackenzie's tracing illustrates 2:1 atrioventricular block.

relaxation) is present. The second portion of the X descent is absent because the blocked A wave is not followed by ventricular systole, so descent of the floor of the right atrium does not occur.

Complete atrioventricular block was described by William Stokes (1846) in his *Observations on Some Cases of Permanently Slow Pulse:*[11]

> A new symptom has appeared, a very remarkable pulsation in the right jugular vein. . . . The number of the reflex pulsations is difficult to be established, but they are more than double the number of the manifest ventricular contractions. About every third pulsation is very strong and sudden and may be seen at a distance; the remaining waves are much less distinct and some very minor ones can also be perceived. The appearance of this patient's neck is very singular, and the pulsation of the veins is of a kind which we have never before witnessed.

This classic description of the jugular pulse in complete heart block is a model of clarity. Co-ordinated atrial activity is more rapid than and is dissociated from ventricular activity that arises from a slow, regular, idioventricular focus (Fig. 4–24). The long diastoles permit identification of the independent A waves which are punctuated by intermittent amplified cannon waves as right atrial contraction fortuitously coincides with right ventricular systole and a closed tricuspid valve (Fig. 4–24). Accordingly, complete heart block is diagnosed in the jugular venous pulse when intermittent cannon A waves occur with smaller independent A waves at a rate faster than the ventricular bradycardia identified by the slow carotid pulse.

VEINS OF THE EXTREMITIES AND THORACIC INLET

Lower Extremities. The physical examination of lower extremity veins seeks chiefly to identify signs of thrombophlebitis (superficial and deep), varicose veins, and chronic venous insufficiency. **Superficial thrombophlebitis** is characterized by an offending thrombus in a vein that can be seen and palpated just beneath the skin, hence

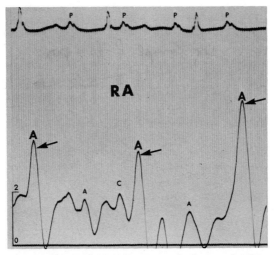

FIGURE 4–24. Right atrial (RA) pressure pulse in complete heart block (the electrocardiogram shows independent P waves). The venous wave form illustrates independent A waves and intermittent cannon A waves *(arrows).*

"superficial." The common sites are the saphenous veins and their tributaries. In the acute state, an indurated, tender cord of varying length is palpable and accompanied by a visible red line along the course of the inflamed vessel. Edema of the extremity is virtually never present. As the acute inflammation subsides, a palpable nontender cord sometimes persists for weeks. Thrombophlebitis usually destroys venous valves, rendering them incompetent when the leg is dependent.

Deep thrombophlebitis typically involves calf veins or iliofemoral veins and may initially escape attention because physical signs (and symptoms) are apt to be scanty early in the course. It is therefore important for the physical examination to seek signs of deep vein thrombophlebitis in clinical settings that heighten suspicion—congestive heart failure, the postpartum period, after major surgery, during protracted debilitating illnesses, and in elderly patients who sit for hours with their legs dependent. Local calf tenderness is often the

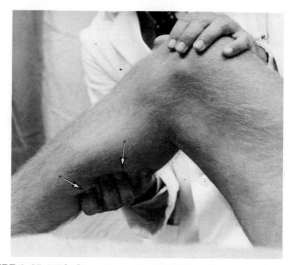

FIGURE 4–25. With the patient supine and knee flexed, the examiner's fingertips gently compress the relaxed calf muscles *(arrow)* against the tibia.

earliest sign. With the patient supine and the knee flexed, the examiner systematically and *gently* compresses the relaxed calf muscles against the tibia. Gentle compression with the fingertips, as shown in Figure 4–25, is preferable to squeezing the calf, a maneuver that can elicit pain in normal subjects. Homans' sign—dorsiflexion of the foot—is far less sensitive than systematic compression of the calf as just described. Homans' sign is unreliable because a positive sign is present in only about 50 per cent of patients with deep vein thrombophlebitis of the calf, and the sign may be elicited in the absence of venous thrombosis because of muscular disorders of the lower extremities. In addition to local tenderness, deep vein thrombosis is generally accompanied by swelling together with increased skin temperature and tissue turgor. Ilio-femoral venous thrombosis is accompanied by tenderness, pain, edema, skin suffusion, increased skin temperature, and visible superficial venous patterns.

Varicose veins represent the most frequent clinical vascular abnormality of the lower extremities. Hippocrates recognized this commonplace disorder 2500 years ago. Nevertheless, varicose veins are often overlooked or underestimated during routine physical examination because the legs are not properly assessed while the patient is standing.

The word "varicose" is derived from the Latin *varicosus*, the adjectival form of *varix*, meaning "a tortuous blood vessel." The plural of varix is *varices*, a term still in general use. Varicose veins, varices, or varicosities vary from cosmetically undesirable but medically unimportant localized clusters of small intracutaneous vessels, to the dramatic, serpentine dilatation shown in Figure 4–26. It is worth underscoring that gravity distends the vessels maximally, so examination in the standing position is obligatory.

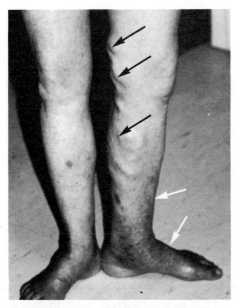

FIGURE 4–26. Varicose veins *(black arrows)* readily seen with the patient standing. The *white arrows* identify swelling and venous stasis in the lower third of the left leg, ankle, and foot. (Courtesy of Dr. Ronald W. Busuttil, Professor of Surgery, UCLA Medical Center.)

Hieronymus Fabricus (1537–1619) described venous valves as "extremely delicate little membranes in the lumen of veins," an observation that is said to have influenced William Harvey's study of the circulation of the blood. Incompetence of venous valves—superficial (saphenous) and deep (iliofemoral)—sets the stage for **chronic venous insufficiency**, the physical signs of which are characteristic. The leg is swollen, and the skin and subcutaneous tissues of the lower third of the leg and ankle—the "stasis areas"—are discolored by brownish pigmentation (Fig. 4–26). Cellulitis, skin erosion, and ulcerations develop especially around the malleoli, more commonly the internal malleolus.

The high systemic venous pressure accompanying right ventricular failure aggravates the distention of varicosities. Tricuspid regurgitation, especially when severe, occasionally imparts systolic pulsations to the varicose veins.

The Upper Extremities. Distention of veins of the dorsa of the hands or antecubital fossae without intrinsic venous disease occurs when central venous pressure is appreciably elevated. Dorsal hand veins are sometimes used to assess central venous pressure. With the patient's trunk adjusted above the horizontal for comfort, the hand under scrutiny is first lowered beneath the sternal angle, without flexing the elbow, until its dorsal veins distend. The arm is then gradually and passively raised while observing the dorsal veins as the hand approaches the level of the sternal angle. Normally, the dorsal hand veins empty at that level when the patient's trunk is 30 to 40 degrees above the horizontal. Persistent distention above that level indicates an elevation of central venous pressure, the height of which is estimated by determining the vertical distance above the angle of Louis at which the dorsal veins visibly collapse. Transmission of systolic pulsations of severe tricuspid regurgitation into dorsal hand veins implies incompetence of the valve of the subclavian vein at the thoracic inlet in the presence of high systemic venous pressure.

Intrinsic disease of veins of the arms and hands is uncommon apart from the sequelae of therapeutic intravenous infusions and injections. The tender, indurated red cord at the site of a heparin lock is a case in point. Not so innocent are the nontender pigmented "main line" streaks, often with palpable cords, that are caused by intravenous drug abuse. The most common sites are antecubital fossae, ventral surfaces of the arms, and dorsa of the hands (see Fig. 2–32).

Thoracic Inlet Veins. Axillary or subclavian thrombophlebitis is rare, but the manifestations result in a relatively typical array of physical signs. Axillary vein thrombophlebitis usually occurs in young patients after trauma to or excessive exertion of the arms. The extremity rapidly becomes swollen (over a period of hours) and assumes a reddish, cyanotic hue. The skin is warm and there is distention of the superficial veins and tenderness in the axilla. When the subclavian vein is the site of thrombophlebitis, tenderness is elicted along its course above the clavicle.

Superior vena caval obstruction—the "superior vena cava syndrome"—is a diagnosis that can be made at the bedside.[12] The deep jugular veins are bilaterally *distended* but *nonpulsatile. Sudden* or *rapid* superior caval obstruction is uncommon. There is dramatic distention of the neck veins in addition to cyanosis and pronounced edema of the face and eyes. *Chronic* obstruction of the superior vena cava is accompanied by suffusion ànd/or cyanosis of the face, neck, and arms, together with dilated, serpentine channels in the neck and arms and over the thorax (collateral flow). Edema of the eyes and face is less pronounced than with acute superior vena caval obstruction.

REFERENCES

1. Mackenzie, J.: The Study of the Pulse, Arterial, Venous and Hepatic, and of the Movements of the Heart. Edinburgh, Young J. Pentland, 1902.
2. Wood, P. W.: Diseases of the Heart and Circulation. Philadelphia, J. B. Lippincott Company, 1956.
3. Potain, P. C. E.: On the movements and sounds that take place in the jugular veins. Bull. Mem. Soc. Med. Hop. Paris 4:3, 1867. *In*

Willius, F. A., and Keys, T. E.: Classics of Cardiology, Vol. 2. Malabar, Florida, Robert E. Krieger Publishing Co., 1983.

4. Hirschfelder, A. D.: Some variations in the form of the venous pulse. Bull. Johns Hopkins Hosp. 18:265, 1907.

5. Wiggers, C. J.: The Pressure Pulses in the Cardiovascular System. London, Longman, Green and Co., 1928.

6. Rondot, E.: Le reflux hepato-jugulaire. Gaz. Hebd. Sc. Med. Bordeaux 19:569, 1898.

7. Pasteur, W.: Note on a new physical sign of tricuspid regurgitation. Lancet 2:524, 1885.

8. Friedreich, N.: Zur diagnose der herzbeutelverwachsungen. Virchows Arch. Pathol. Anat. 29:296, 1864.

9. Kussmaul, A.: Uber schwielige mediastino-pericarditis und den paradoxen pulse. Berl. Klin. Wochenschr. 10:433, 1873.

10. Gibson, A. G.: The significance of a hitherto undescribed wave in the jugular pulse. Lancet 2:1380, 1907.

11. Stokes, W.: Observations on some cases of permanently slow pulse. Dublin Q. J. Med. Sci. 2:73, 1846.

12. Parish, J. M., Marschke, R. F., Dines, D. E., and Lee, R. E.: Etiologic considerations in superior vena cava syndrome. Mayo Clin. Proc. 56:407, 1981.

THE MOVEMENTS OF THE HEART— PERCUSSION, PALPATION, AND OBSERVATION

Egyptian physicians and priests employed the technique of palpation, and there is little doubt that palpation was part of the physical examination in ancient Greece (Fig. 5–1) and in the Middle Ages. William Harvey's treatise (1628) is commonly referred to by its short title *De Motu Cordis*—Of the Motion of the Heart.[1] In Chapter II, Harvey dealt with the motions of the heart imparted to the chest wall: "In the first place, then, when the chest of a living animal is laid open and the capsule that immediately surrounds the heart is slit up or removed, the organ is seen now to move, now to be at rest. . . ."[1] Harvey then made it clear that the movements of the heart could be identified on the intact chest wall, stating, " . . . the heart is erected, and rises upward to a point, so that at this time it strikes against the breast and the pulse is felt externally."[1] Laënnec (1819) not only defined the location and size of the apex beat but described movements conveyed to the chest wall by both left *and* right ventricles.

> In a healthy person of moderate fullness and whose heart is well proportioned, the pulsation of this organ is only perceived in the cardiac region, that is, in the space comprised between the carti-

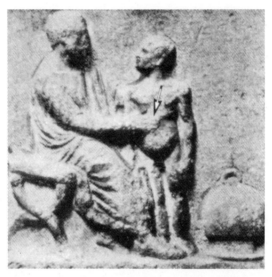

FIGURE 5–1. Greek bas-relief showing the physician Jason using palpation *(arrow)* in the examination of a young patient. (Modified from Castiglioni A.: A History of Medicine. New York, Alfred A. Knopf, 1947.)

lages of the fifth and seventh ribs, and under the lower end of the sternum. The motions of the left cavities of the heart are chiefly perceptible in the former position, those of the right cavities in the latter. This is so much the case, that, in disease of one side of the heart only, the pulsation in these two situations gives quite different results. When the sternum is short, the pulsations extend to the epigastrium.[2]

James Mackenzie's *The Study of the Pulse* (1902) contains a chapter on "The Movements of the Heart in Health and in Disease"[3] that represents a landmark in understanding cardiac motion imparted to the thorax. The message is still relevant. Practically all important precordial movements transmitted by a beating heart can be palpated and seen by an experienced clinician. It is exciting to witness the useful diagnostic conclusions that can be drawn from these observations.

Percussion retains a place in the physical examination of the heart and circulation, albeit an abridged one relative to the older art of palpation. Recall that Auenbrugger inaugurated the modern art of physical diagnosis with his discovery of percussion, observing that the level of fluid in his native wine casks could be ascertained by thumping (Fig. 5–2). Referring specifically to the heart, Auenbrugger wrote, " . . . over the space occupied by the heart, the sound loses part of its usual clearness, and becomes dull. The whole sternum yields as distinct a sound as the sides of the chest, except in the cardiac region where it is somewhat duller."[4] I generally begin with percussion, followed by observation and palpation.

PERCUSSION

Percussion is best achieved through the intermediary of the bone of the examiner's applied finger, which serves to amplify the response. To elicit the percussion note, the entire length of the middle finger of one hand is applied firmly to the site under study while the dorsum of that digit is percussed (tapped) by the tip of the arched

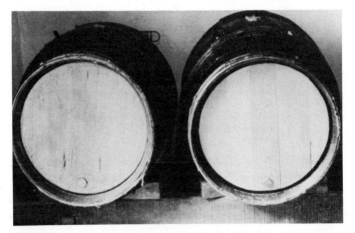

FIGURE 5–2. Leopold Auenbrugger witnessed his father's practice of percussing wine barrels (shown here) to determine the level of their contents. The observation led to " . . . a new sign which I have discovered. . . . This consists of the Percussion of the human thorax."[4]

middle finger of the other hand using the wrist as the fulcrum.

Information derived from percussion falls into two categories: (1) determination of visceral situs—heart, stomach, and liver, and (2) the less important approximations of the left and right cardiac borders. Before beginning the physical examination of the heart per se, the location of cardiac and hepatic dullness and gastric tympany must be established, especially but not only in infants, children, and young adults. Situs solitus with levocardia (normal positions) is established at the bedside by percussing gastric tympany on the left and hepatic dullness on the right, while comparative percussion to the left and right of the sternum identifies cardiac dullness on the left (levocardia). If the tympanitic note from the stomach is not clearly evident, the patient should be instructed to inhale and swallow a few times (aerophagia), a maneuver that generally resolves the problem. An infant swallows air when given an empty bottle to suck.

Situs inversus with dextrocardia (mirror image) is the reverse of the above, with gastric tympany on the right, hepatic dullness on the left, and cardiac dullness to the right of the sternum (Fig. 5–3). Ninety-five per cent of patients with mirror image dextrocardia have no coexisting congenital heart disease, but unless situs inversus with dextrocardia is identified, symptoms accompanying *acquired* heart disease can be misleading. The pain of myocardial ischemia is likely to be *right* precordial with radiation to the right arm. Acute cholecystitis presents with pain in the left upper quadrant, and acute appendicitis presents with pain in the left lower quadrant.

Apart from identification of visceral situs, percussion competes poorly with palpation and observation of the precordium as described below. With few exceptions, observation and palpation provide all information available by percussion and much more. However, percussion is sometimes useful in approximating the position of the left cardiac border when the apex cannot be confidently identified by palpation. In the presence of a large pericardial effusion, cardiac dullness is occasionally elicited lateral to the left ventricular impulse. A very large peri-

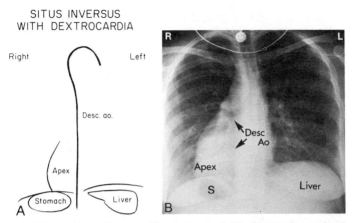

SITUS INVERSUS
WITH DEXTROCARDIA

FIGURE 5–3. *A,* Schematic illustration and *(B)* chest radiograph of dextrocardia in situs inversus. At the bedside, abdominal visceral position is established by percussing the stomach (S) on the right and the liver on the left. Cardiac dullness (apex) on the right establishes dextrocardia.

cardial effusion can cause dullness over the sternum and even to the right of the sternum. A dilated right atrium may also cause dullness to the right of the sternum, and a giant *left* atrium may form the right lower cardiac border and cause overlying dullness to percussion.

OBSERVATION AND PALPATION (Table 5–1)

Topographic Anatomy of the Heart and Designation of Precordial Sites. Diagnostic conclusions based upon observation and palpation presuppose knowledge of the

TABLE 5–1. Information from Observation and Palpation

Systolic movements of the ventricles
Diastolic movements of the ventricles
Systolic movements of the great arteries
Systolic movements of the atria
Palpable heart sounds
Palpable murmurs (thrills)

topographic anatomy of the underlying cardiac and vascular structures that impart movements or vibrations to the chest wall. These chest wall sites should be referred to by simple, unambiguous descriptive terms.

The chief topographic areas for routine observation and palpation in patients with normal visceral positions (levocardia in situs solitus) are the cardiac apex and the sternal borders (left and right; lower, middle, and upper). The examination can then be refined by palpation in individual parasternal interspaces, in the subxiphoid region, and over the sternoclavicular junctions.

In the normal heart, the apex is on the left and is occupied by an anatomic *left* ventricle (Figs. 5–4 and 5–5). The anatomic *right* ventricle is anterior and inferior (Figs. 5–4 and 5–5). The inflow or sinus portion of the right ventricle underlies the fourth and fifth left intercostal spaces, while the outflow portion (infundibulum) underlies the third left interspace. The main pulmonary artery (pulmonary trunk) lies beneath the second left interspace (Fig. 5–5). The border of the right atrium is

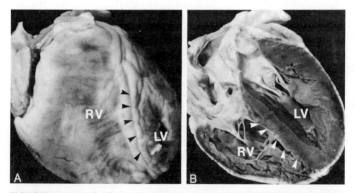

FIGURE 5–4. *A,* The heart in its in situ position. The left ventricle (LV) occupies the apex and is separated from the anterior right ventricle (RV) by the interventricular sulcus *(arrowheads).* (B) Sagittal section through the heart in its in situs position showing the right ventricle inferior, anterior, and to the right of the left ventricle *(arrowheads—*ventricular septum). Labels mine. (Reprinted with permission from Anderson, R. F., and Becker, A. E.: Cardiac Anatomy. London, Gower Medical Publishing, 1980.)

NORMAL

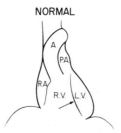

FIGURE 5–5. Topographic anatomy of the normal heart. *Arrow* points to the interventricular sulcus. The left ventricle (LV) occupies the apex. The body of the right ventricle (RV) is anterior, underlying the lower left sternal border (fourth and fifth interspaces); the infundibulum underlies the mid-left sternal edge (third interspace); and the main pulmonary artery (PA) is beneath the second left interspace. The aortic root (A) is convex to the right of the sternum in the second interspace, and the right atrial border is just to the right of the lower sternal edge. Compare to Figure 5–4.

just lateral to the lower right sternal edge, and the aortic root (ascending aorta) is convex to the right of the sternum at the level of the second right interspace (Fig. 5–5). The left atrium is not border-forming because it is a posterior structure, except for its appendage, which underlies the third left interspace.

Methodology and Technique of Observation and Palpation. The examination should be performed with the clinician standing or sitting comfortably to the right of the bedside or examining table. In older children and adults, the patient's trunk should be elevated about 30 degrees above the horizontal, first supine and then in a partial left lateral decubitus position (Fig. 5–6). Infants are, as a rule, examined supine but can sometimes be turned into a partial left lateral decubitus position. In adult females, large breasts should be retracted. The patient can assist in this maneuver when the examiner's hands are occupied with both palpation and timing (see below).

The palmar surfaces of the hand—fingertips, distal metacarpals, or the "heel" of the hand—and the amount of pressure applied vary according to what is anticipated from palpation and according to the precordial site under

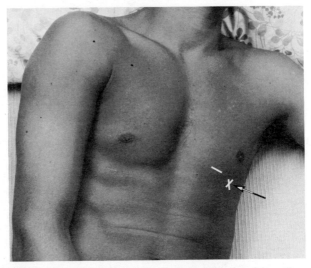

FIGURE 5–6. Partial left lateral decubitus position for observation and palpation of the left ventricle. The lateral mark (+, *arrow*) is over the left ventricle, which moves anterior during systole, while the right ventricle (medial mark) retracts (−). Retraction begins at the interventricular sulcus (see Figs. 5–4 and 5–5). The carotid pulse can be palpated for timing purposes, as shown in Figure 5–7.

assessment. Detection of relatively high-frequency events (thrills, ejection sounds, prominent first and second heart sounds) benefits from relatively firm pressure using the palmar surface of the distal metacarpals. With this exception, virtually all other information from palpation—the movements of the heart—is best identified by using the pads of the fingertips, which serve not only to detect precordial movement but more precisely to localize it. The "heel" of the hand firmly applied to the left sternal border is a method for sensing relatively obvious, diffuse systolic movement (see later). However, the impulses in this area, especially when subtle and localized, are more readily detected by applying the fingertips between the ribs, as shown in Figure 5–7 and as described in detail later. In infants, a single fingertip suffices (Fig. 5–8).

Subxiphoid palpation should be routine because, as Laënnec pointed out, "pulsations extend to the epigas-

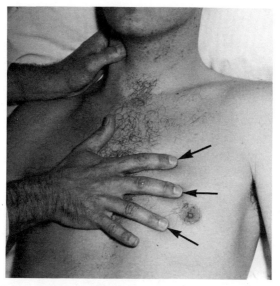

FIGURE 5–7. Palpation of the anterior wall of the right ventricle by applying the tips of three fingers in the third, fourth, and fifth interspaces, left sternal edge *(arrows),* during full held exhalation. The carotid can be used for timing purposes as shown. Patient is supine with the trunk elevated 30 degrees.

trium.'' Palpation at this site is best achieved in older children and adults by resting the flat of the hand upon the epigastrium while directing the tip of the index finger upward and to the left to make contact with the right ventricular impulse as it descends during held inspiration (Fig. 5–9A). In infants, subxiphoid palpation is best achieved with the tip of the little finger (Fig. 5–9B).

The respiratory position during precordial palpation is important. Held deep inspiration in older children or adults improves detection of the subxiphoid right ventricular impulse and minimizes mistaking this impulse for the aortic pulsation, which is palpated on the palmar surface of the fingers during held *expiration* (Fig. 5–10). Held expiration also improves detection of subtle systolic and diastolic movements of the left ventricle (apex) and of the right ventricle (left parasternal edge). Thrills, with

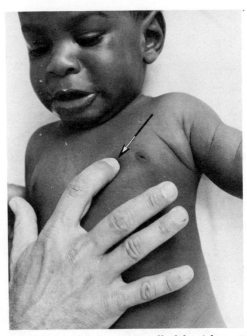

FIGURE 5–8. Palpation of the anterior wall of the right ventricle in an infant. A single fingertip *(arrow)* is applied to the mid-left sternal edge.

few exceptions, are more readily identified during full held expiration as the distal metacarpals are firmly applied to the area of interest. More precise localization of thrills is then achieved by relatively firm application of the fingertips at specific localized sites.

Before beginning systematic palpation, it is sometimes useful to *observe* the precordium for movements that are obvious at a glance. During or after palpation, *detailed observation* serves to clarify subtle movements. These movements can be enhanced by applying pen marks on the skin at the site under observation (see Fig. 5–6) and by using a source of oblique illumination (pocket flashlight). The examiner should then look *across* the chest *tangentially* rather than from above. Parasternal movements are sometimes best seen when the examiner looks

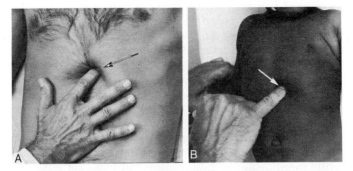

FIGURE 5–9. *A,* Subxiphoid palpation of the inferior wall of the right ventricle in an adult. The tip of the index finger *(arrow)* is directed upward and to the left, palpating the right ventricle as it descends during held inspiration. *B,* In infants, subcostal palpation of the right ventricle is best achieved using the tip of the little finger *(arrow)*.

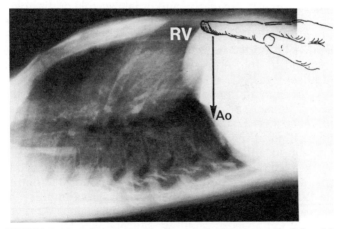

FIGURE 5–10. Subxiphoid palpation of the inferior wall of the right ventricle (RV) with the relative position of the abdominal aorta (Ao) shown by the *arrow.*

upward from the patient's feet. Precordial *retraction* is more readily seen than palpated, whereas outward displacement is more readily palpated than seen.

The *timing of precordial movements*—observed or palpated—can be achieved by using the carotid pulse (see Fig. 5–7) or the heart sounds as references. My preference in older children and adults is to apply the thumb of the left hand to the carotid pulse while observing or palpating the precordium with the right hand (see Fig. 5–7). Alternatively, the stethoscope can be held in place with the left hand, freeing the right hand for palpation or observation of precordial movements. It is sometimes useful to observe systolic movement imparted to the stethoscope while monitoring the first and second heart sounds. This point recalls Laënnec's comment on the "shock or impulse" communicated to his wooden stethoscopic cylinder as it was applied to the cardiac apex.

In assessing the movements of the heart imparted to the chest wall, it is necessary to determine the topographic location of a given impulse as well as its timing in the cardiac cycle (early, mid or late systole or diastole), its duration (how much of the cardiac cycle the impulse occupies), its displacement characteristics (vigor of movement, amplitude, and contour), and the maximum area occupied by the impulse (especially the left ventricular impulse).

Apart from and in addition to the location (situs) of the heart, stomach, and liver, a number of other variables influence the position of the heart and the pulsations transmitted to the chest wall. Among these variables are body build and thoracic configuration (see Chapter 2). Scoliosis to the right rotates the heart leftward on its long axis; pectus excavatum shifts the heart to the left, altering the position of the normal left ventricular impulse. A decrease in anteroposterior chest dimensions (loss of thoracic kyphosis or shallow, saucer-shaped pectus excavatum) increases contact of the right ventricle with the anterior chest wall. Ascites or pregnancy elevates the diaphragm and with it the heart, whereas a tall, thin habitus has the opposite effect. Eventration of the left hemidiaphragm (infants) shifts the heart to the right, often dramatically so.

Normal Precordial Movement. Palpation and observation of normal precordial movement assumes awareness of the characteristics of left and right ventricular impulses. Systolic movements imparted by the ventricles should be designated according to which ventricle—left or right—is causing the impulse. The term "point of maximum impulse" (PMI) is imprecise and is best replaced by a term that reflects the origin of the impulse or, lacking that, simple topographic location (apical, parasternal, etc.).

At birth, the comparatively thick-walled anterior and inferior right ventricle is responsible for normal systolic precordial movement palpated at the mid to lower left sternal edge and in the subxiphoid region. The movement is gentle, tapping, and unsustained. Separate systolic movement by the left ventricle cannot, as a rule, be identified even when the infant is turned into a partial left lateral decubitus position. Elevation of the baby's trunk in an infant's seat improves perception of the normal subxiphoid right ventricular impulse as the heart descends. During normal development, the left ventricle outgrows the right, so that in older infants, children, and adults of average body build, the only normal precordial systolic impulse is left ventricular. However, in some slightly built patients, and in the presence of diminished anteroposterior chest dimensions (loss of thoracic kyphosis, shallow pectus excavatum), a normal, gentle, unsustained right ventricular impulse persists at the mid to lower left sternal edge, but seldom in the subxiphoid region.

During left ventricular isometric contraction and early ejection (Fig. 5–11), the left ventricle rotates on its long axis so that its apex moves toward the chest wall (Fig. 5–6). James Mackenzie's comment is relevant: "With the onset of ventricular systole a great change takes place in the position of the left ventricle. The muscle hardens and contracts upon its contents, and at the same time the heart twists round, so that the hardened apex projects forward, pressing against the chest wall. . . ."[3] The nor-

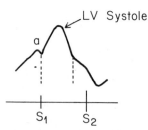

FIGURE 5–11. Apex cardiogram illustrating the duration of a normal left ventricular (LV) systolic impulse, which returns to baseline before the last third of systole. The "a" crest represents presystolic LV filling in response to atrial contraction. S_1 = first heart sound; S_2 = second heart sound.

mal left ventricular impulse consists of a localized, gentle, unsustained anterior apical systolic movement with retraction medial to the interventricular sulcus (see Figs. 5–4 to 5–6). Retraction occurs because the anterior right ventricle is drawn away from the chest wall during systole. The normal zone of medial retraction is relatively localized (see Fig. 5–6), i.e., not extending to the left sternal edge. The normal left ventricular systolic impulse is also localized, generally to one interspace, and normally occupies an area less than 3 cm in diameter in adults.

A horizontal supine position provides the lowest yield for detecting a left ventricular impulse, especially when the impulse is normal or nearly so. Accordingly, I generally begin palpation in older children and adults in a partial left lateral decubitus position with trunk elevated approximately 30 degrees above the horizontal. This position permits identification of the left ventricular impulse in virtually all patients in whom the left ventricle occupies the apex, especially when palpation is performed during held exhalation. Obesity and emphysema are exceptions. The left ventricular impulse should initially be sought with the apposed pads of several fingers, shifting the overlying skin in search of the localized tap, which is then palpated with the tips of the fingers (cupping the hand) and finally, and more precisely, with the tip of a single finger, generally the first or second (Fig. 5–

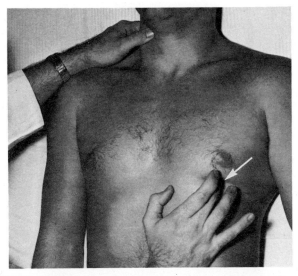

FIGURE 5–12. Palpation of the left ventricular impulse with a fingertip *(arrow)*. The patient's trunk is 30 degrees above the horizontal. The examiner's right thumb palpates the carotid pulse for timing purposes.

12). These maneuvers require just enough time and concentration to attune the examiner and heighten tactile sensitivity. Once anterior ventricular movement is palpated, medial retraction must be established. To achieve this, the palpating fingertip, without being lifted, can be moved medially with the overlying skin, a maneuver that results in loss of the impulse because the medial retraction is not readily palpated. The fingertip can then be returned to the palpable impulse while the examiner *observes* medial retraction. Marking the skin (see Fig. 5–6) and use of a tangential light source as described earlier adds refinement to the observation of an anterior apical impulse with medial retraction, confirming that the impulse is left ventricular.

When the left ventricular impulse is not palpable in the left lateral decubitus position despite a meticulous search, percussion can be used to estimate the location of the left cardiac border. Further palpation at that site might then detect the elusive left ventricular movement. The *location* of the left ventricular impulse, is by convention, judged relative to the midclavicular line or by the distance of the impulse from the left sternal edge, and by the interspace in which the impulse is palpable. Location should also take into account the patient's age and thoracic size and shape. The normal left ventricular impulse in the supine position (with the thorax elevated as described above) is generally located in the fifth intercostal space at or medial to the midclavicular line (Fig. 5–12). In infants and in adults with short, stocky chests, the impulse is often in the fourth left interspace. In tall, thin persons with linear positions of the heart, the left ventricular impulse is sometimes sufficiently close to the left sternal edge to prompt a mistaken impression of a *right* ventricular impulse. Re-examination in the left lateral decubitus position avoids this error by permitting identification of the telltale anterior displacement of the left ventricle with retraction medial to the interventricular sulcus.

Although the left lateral decubitus position has the advantage of increasing the probability of palpating the left ventricular impulse so that its displacement characteristics can be assessed, the *location* of the impulse in the lateral decubitus does not accurately reflect left ventricular size (enlargment). If the impulse remains palpable as the patient returns to the supine position, its location can then be reassessed.

The left ventricular impulse is difficult to identify in the sitting position. In the occasional patient who is apt to be examined while sitting (neuromuscular disease, for example), the impulse, if palpable, can be relatively confidently related to the landmarks described above for the supine position.

Mackenzie reassured us that in assessing the displacement characteristics of the left ventricular impulse, "A cardiogram *(graphic record, sic)* is not nearly so instructive as the physical examination of the apex beat. The position, size and strength of the apex beat can be far better appreciated by the palpating hand."[3] The *duration* of the left ventricular impulse is a feature that distinguishes normal from abnormal. Normally, there is a single outward (anterior) movement during isometric contraction and during early ejection. The movement returns to baseline before the last third of systole (Fig. 5–11). The maximum area occupied by the normal left ventricular impulse—its *size*—is less than 3 cm in diameter in adults. This is so even in the left lateral decubitus position.

Velocity and amplitude of a normal left ventricular impulse vary somewhat according to relaxation or anxiety of the patient. In anxious patients, there is often an increase in both the velocity and amplitude of the impulse, but *not* in its duration or area. The relative ease with which a normal but hyperkinetic left ventricular impulse is palpated invites the mistaken notion that the duration and area of the impulse are also increased.

Abnormal Systolic Movements of the Left Ventricle. An abnormal left ventricular impulse can be characterized according to its location (including an ectopic location), displacement characteristics, and contour. The systolic impulse of an enlarged left ventricle is not only displaced laterally but is usually palpated in the sixth rather than the fifth intercostal space because the ribs slant upward as the anterior axillary line is approached. The sixth interspace at the anterior axillary line is at the same horizontal level as the fifth interspace at the midclavicular line. In addition, dilatation of the left ventricle (an increase in internal dimensions) tends to displace the apex *inferiorly* as well as laterally (Fig. 5–13).

An "*ectopic*" left ventricular impulse occupies a site that is not anticipated in normally positioned (situs solitus) hearts. The most common site of an ectopic impulse is *above* and *medial* to the expected location of the left ventricular impulse. The ectopic segment—often as readily seen as palpated—is usually caused by the anterior wall dyskinesis of ischemic heart disease.

Prolonged (sustained) *duration* of a relatively normally located left ventricular systolic impulse is typical of pressure hypertrophy with increased wall thickness but normal internal dimensions. Laënnec made the point: "The more intense the hypertrophia, the longer the time the impulse is perceptible. . . ."[2] A sustained left ventric-

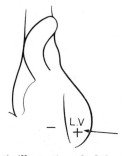

FIGURE 5–13. Schematic illustration of a left ventricular (LV) impulse that is displaced to the left and inferiorly *(arrow)*. When displacement is due to *volume* overload, a hyperkinetic LV systolic impulse (+) is accompanied by exaggerated medial retraction (−).

ular impulse proceeds into the latter third of systole, approaching the second heart sound when timed by auscultation, in contrast to the normal impulse illustrated in Figure 5–11.

Abnormal *velocity* and *amplitude* of a left ventricular impulse can be graded from hypokinetic (decreased) to hyperkinetic (markedly increased). Reduced velocity and amplitude (hypokinesis) of the left ventricular impulse in a patient of normal body build is a sign of decreased contractility, especially when accompanied by a laterally displaced impulse (dilated cardiomyopathy, for example). When the left ventricle is hypokinetic and *markedly* displaced laterally and inferiorly, its impulse may initially be missed because the examiner palpates too far medially. Percussion in the supine position prevents this error and directs attention to the true lateral cardiac border, which may extend to the posterior axillary line. A hypokinetic left ventricular impulse (low velocity and amplitude of systolic motion) is generally accompanied by reduced velocity and amplitude of medial retraction, making detection more difficult. A normally located (or ectopic) left ventricular impulse of *increased* amplitude and duration (though not of velocity) is a feature of postmyocardial infarction dyskinesis (Fig. 5–14) but may occur transiently during a bout of angina pectoris. This prolonged systolic impulse of regional dyskinesis is really "paradoxic" because it bulges abnormally during mid to late systole (Fig. 5–14), at a time when normal, earlier anterior systolic movement has ceased (see Fig. 5–11).

The maximum area occupied by a normal left ventricular systolic impulse in an adult of average body build is less than 3 cm in diameter, proportionately less in infants and children. An impulse in excess of 3 cm in diameter in adults is good evidence of concentric hypertrophy of systemic hypertension or aortic stenosis or of left ventricular enlargement (increased end-diastolic volume). In the absence of concentric left ventricular hypertrophy, an increase in the maximum *area* occupied by the impulse is more reliable evidence of left ventricular enlargement than the *location* of the impulse relative to the midclavicular line.

The *contour* of the left ventricular impulse is, as a rule, single whether the impulse is otherwise normal or not. However, a *double* systolic impulse is sometimes palpable in hypertrophic obstructive cardiomyopathy (Fig. 5–15). Identification of this double systolic impulse requires

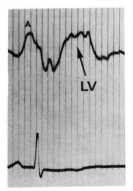

FIGURE 5–14. Apex cardiogram showing sustained apical dyskinesis (left ventricular impulse of prolonged duration, *arrow*) in a patient with a Q wave anterior myocardial infarction. The impulse was palpated in the fifth interspace just beyond the midclavicular line and was preceded by prominent presystolic distention (A). Compare to Figure 5–11.

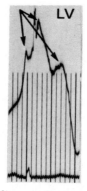

FIGURE 5–15. Apex cardiogram from a patient with hypertrophic obstructive cardiomyopathy. There is a triple left ventricular (LV) impulse caused, in sequence, by presystolic and double systolic movements *(arrows).*

a reference for timing, either the carotid pulse (see Fig. 5–7) or the heart sounds.

When the left ventricle occupies the cardiac apex but the apex *retracts* in systole, the cause is usually chronic constrictive pericarditis.[5] Retraction is usually most pronounced at the apex but may extend as far as the left sternal edge.

Abnormal Systolic Movements of the Right Ventricle. Laënnec was aware of an abnormal right ventricular impulse when he applied his stethoscopic cylinder to the precordium: "The contractions of the heart, as explored by the cylinder, gave the same results nearly, whether the hypertrophia be on the right or the left side; only in the former case, the shock of the heart's action is greater at the bottom of the sternum. ..."[2] James Mackenzie identified and recorded the epigastric impulse of the right ventricle and distinguished it from the impulse of the abdominal aorta (see Fig. 5–10). Mackenzie wrote, "At the postmortem examination a needle pushed through the epigastrium, at the place where the tracing was obtained, was found to have penetrated the right ventricle."[3] By contrast, " . . . epigastric pulsation, due to the abdominal aorta, presents quite a different character from that due to a dilated right ventricle. . . ." (see Fig. 5–10).

For assessment of right ventricular systolic movement, the examiner stands or sits to the right, and the patient is examined supine, with the thorax horizontal or elevated 30 degrees. In situs solitus, the anatomic right ventricle is anterior and inferior (see Fig. 5–4) and topographically behind the left sternal edge. Its inflow portion underlies the mid to lower left sternal edge (fourth and fifth intercostal spaces), while its outflow portion (infundibulum) lies behind the third interspace. Accordingly, the areas potentially in contact with the anterior chest wall are relatively greater in contrast to the limited potential contact of the left ventricle with the chest wall. The inferior portion of the right ventricle (see Fig. 5–4) transmits its impulse to the subxiphoid region, which is accessible to palpation (see Fig. 5–9). In patients old enough to cooperate, palpation of the right ventricle in the subxiphoid area should be carried out during held *inspiration*, whereas palpation of the right ventricle at the left sternal edge should be carried out during held *exhalation*.

Age and thoracic configuration materially influence access to the right ventricle. In infants, the right ventricle is responsible for the normal precordial impulse as described earlier. In older children and adults with slight body builds or decreased anteroposterior chest dimensions (loss of thoracic kyphosis, shallow pectus excavatum), an intrinsically normal right ventricle increases its contact with the anterior chest wall, producing a gentle, brief left parasternal impulse. Conversely, an *increase* in anteroposterior chest dimensions (pulmonary emphysema) serves to reduce or abolish contact of the right ventricle with the anterior chest wall even when the chamber is enlarged, so its impulse may not be palpable at the left sternal edge. Subxiphoid palpation (see Figs. 5–9A and 5–10) provides an important alternative, especially because hyperinflation of the emphysematous lungs lowers the diaphragm and with it the inferior wall of the right ventricle.

Observation plays an important but lesser role than

palpation in assessing right ventricular systolic impulses; percussion is of little or no value. Two methods of *right ventricular palpation* are recommended, as already briefly described. The heel of the hand can be applied firmly to the left sternal edge during full expiration, keeping the fingers elevated while sensing the systolic impulse and observing the motion of the hand imparted by right ventricular contraction. This technique is relatively insensitive in detecting subtle systolic movement and does not localize the impulses so derived. A more refined method employs several fingertips applied simultaneously and in parallel in the third, fourth, and fifth intercostal spaces during held expiration (see Fig. 5–7). The free left hand is used for timing with the right carotid pulse as a reference (see Fig. 5–7) or by applying the stethoscope to the chest for identification of the first and second heart sounds. This method of palpation not only permits detection of gentle right ventricular systolic impulses but localizes the movements to the inflow portion (fourth and fifth intercostal spaces) or to the infundibulum or outflow portion (third interspace). In infants, palpation along the left sternal border is best accomplished with the tip of a single finger during active breathing (see Fig. 5–8) or during very brief arrested respiration induced by pinching the nostrils while the infant sucks on a nipple or pacifier.

The normal impulse of the right ventricle in older children and adults is characterized by a brief, gentle, early systolic outward movement (not palpable in persons of average body build), followed immediately by retraction—movement away from the chest wall—that occupies the rest of systole. In older children or adults of average body build, the right ventricle is not normally palpable.

Right ventricular systolic anterior movement is accompanied by *lateral* retraction in the region of the interventricular sulcus (see Fig. 5–4). When the right ventricle is *appreciably* enlarged, it occupies the apex, displacing the left ventricle, which no longer makes contact with the chest wall and therefore imparts no precordial impulse (Fig. 5–16). In this setting, right ventricular systolic movement extends from the left sternal edge to the cardiac

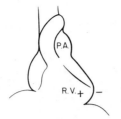

FIGURE 5–16. Schematic illustration of an enlarged right ventricle (RV) that displaces the left ventricle from the apex. The positive (+) right ventricular systolic impulse extends to the apex, which retracts (−). A dilated main pulmonary artery (PA) underlies the second left interspace.

apex which retracts (Fig. 5–16). Mackenzie described these points in admirable detail:

> Accepting the usual clinical definition of the apex beat being the lowest and outermost part of the heart's impulse, a totally different form of beat is found when the right ventricle causes this movement. In certain cases of dilatation of the right heart, nearly the whole anterior aspect of the heart is composed of the right auricle and ventricle, the left ventricle forming a mere strip of the lateral border. This portion of the left ventricle is situated so far back that it is covered by the lungs and does not reach the chest wall. Therefore, the lowest and outermost part of the heart in contact with the chest wall is the right ventricle. . . . In place of the outward thrust during systole, as in the apex beat due to the left ventricle, there is drawing in of the tissues.[3]

The abnormal systolic anterior movement of the right ventricle with lateral retraction can be highlighted by marking the chest wall, as shown in Figure 5–17. To confirm that the right ventricle occupies the apex, *observation* of movement becomes important because lateral retraction is better seen than palpated.

Characterization of the right ventricular impulse, in addition to timing and location described above, includes contour, velocity, amplitude, and duration of movement. The *contour* of a right ventricular impulse, whether normal or abnormal, is single rather than double. Persistence of the gentle, brief, normal neonatal right ventricular impulse is a feature of Fallot's tetralogy, in which the right ventricle continues to function as a systemic cham-

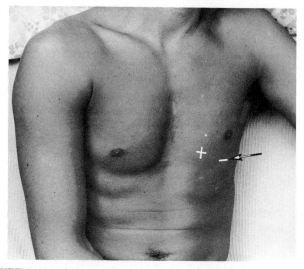

FIGURE 5–17. When an enlarged right ventricle occupies the apex, a positive systolic impulse (+) is palpated from sternal edge to apex, and the apex retracts (−, *arrow*). A separate left ventricular impulse cannot be palpated, even in the left lateral decubitus position. Compare to Figure 5–16.

ber as it does in the fetus and newborn. It is the patient's age and not the displacement characteristics of the right ventricular impulse that make it abnormal. The right ventricular impulse in Fallot's tetralogy is confined to the fourth and fifth intercostal spaces and is not present in the third interspace. This is so because infundibular pulmonic stenosis assigns the elevated right ventricular systolic pressure to the body or inflow portion of the chamber. A right ventricular impulse extending to the *third* interspace means that the systolic pressure is elevated in the outflow *and* inflow portions, as in pulmonic valve stenosis or pulmonary hypertension. Marked to severe elevation of right ventricular systolic pressure with intact ventricular septum is accompanied by an impulse that is increased in amplitude *and* duration from the third to the fifth intercostal space as well as in the subxiphoid area.

A right ventricular impulse characterized by a modest increase in velocity and amplitude, but no increase in duration, is a feature of the *volume* overload of mild to moderate tricuspid regurgitation. At the other end of the spectrum is the dramatic right ventricular impulse accompanying the large left-to-right shunt of an uncomplicated ostium secundum atrial septal defect. These left parasternal and subxiphoid impulses can be tumultuous and the apical retraction exaggerated. Although the impulse is considerably increased in velocity and amplitude, there is comparatively little or no increase in its duration.

In assessing right ventricular systolic movement as described above, *intrinsically* abnormal motion must be distinguished from movement imparted to an otherwise normal right ventricle when the chamber is displaced anteriorly during left ventricular systole. The most common example is mitral regurgitation (Fig. 5–18). The left atrium is a posterior chamber, lying behind the heart and in front of the rigid vertebral column. An enlarged left atrium moves the heart forward, so an otherwise normal right ventricle comes into contact with the anterior chest wall. In addition, mitral regurgitation causes a phasic systolic increase in volume of the large left atrium, producing systolic anterior parasternal movement (Fig. 5–18). The systolic impulse is relatively late because the left ventricle must first contract and provide the regurgitant volume that expands the left atrium and moves the heart forward. The late systolic timing of the impulse is best established in relation to the first heart sound, but timing is sometimes possible by simultaneously palpating the left ventricular impulse while observing or palpating the parasternal systolic movement.

Anterior systolic movement of a normal right ventricle can be caused by certain regional wall motion abnormalities of the *left* ventricle. Dyskinetic motion of the ventricular septum during angina pectoris displaces the right ventricle forward and results in a transient left parasternal impulse that disappears promptly with relief of angina. Post–myocardial infarction dyskinesis of the ventricular septum is analogous but results in persistent systolic anterior displacement of the right ventricle. In mitral

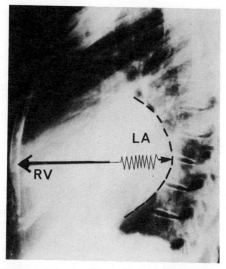

FIGURE 5–18. Lateral chest radiograph in a patient with severe mitral regurgitation and a large left atrium (LA), which displaces the right ventricle (RV) anteriorly and increases its contact with the chest wall. Systolic expansion of the left atrium moves the heart forward with each left ventricular systole *(large arrow)*, rendering the right ventricle palpable.

stenosis, a large left atrium may displace the right ventricle anteriorly and exaggerate *intrinsic* pulsations of that chamber (pulmonary hypertension).

Biventricular Systolic Movements. A pure *left* ventricular impulse causes apical systolic anterior movement with medial retraction (see Fig. 5–6). A pure *right* ventricular systolic impulse causes left parasternal anterior movement with lateral retraction (see Fig. 5–16 and 5–17). When *both* ventricles impart systolic impulses to the precordium, the apical left ventricular impulse and the parasternal right ventricular impulse are separated by a zone of retraction that represents the plane of the interventricular sulcus (see Figs. 5–4 and 5–19).

Mid-Diastolic Movements of Ventricles. Passive filling of the ventricles occurs as atrial pressures rise sufficiently to open the mitral and tricuspid valves. Abnormally rapid

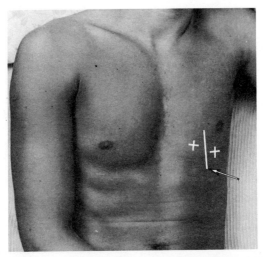

FIGURE 5–19. Biventricular systolic movements of the ventricles with anterior displacement (+) of both right *and* left ventricles separated by a zone of retraction along the interventricular sulcus *(arrow)*. The patient is in a partial left lateral decubitus position.

atrioventricular flow and/or abnormal diastolic properties of the recipient ventricle impart to that chamber a brief, distinct mid-diastolic movement that can be palpated and sometimes seen (Fig. 5–20). The auscultatory counterpart of this movement is an abnormal third heart sound that may be more readily palpated than heard (see Chapter 6). Normal (physiologic) third heart sounds are, for all practical purposes, not palpable.

Detection of mid-diastolic ventricular movement requires attention to the patient's position and phase of respiration and to the technique of palpation and observation. With the thorax elevated 30 degrees above horizontal, the patient is turned into the left lateral decubitus position if the left ventricle is the focus of attention. A mid-diastolic left ventricular impulse that goes unnoticed in the supine position may be relatively obvious in the left lateral decubitus. Once the left ventricle is identified, its impulse should be palpated with a single finger (see Fig. 5–12) while the breath is held in full but comfortable

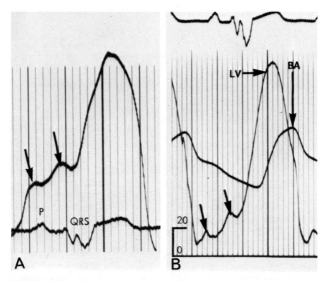

FIGURE 5–20. *A,* Apex cardiogram in a patient with aortic valve stenosis and left ventricular failure. *Arrows* point to mid-diastolic *and* presystolic distention. *B,* Left ventricular (LV) and brachial arterial (BA) pulses in the same patient showing mid-diastolic and presystolic movements *(arrows).* The systolic gradient is also shown.

exhalation. The tactile sensation imparted by mid-diastolic movement varies from bare perceptibility to an obvious impact (Fig. 5–20). A case in point is chronic severe mitral regurgitation with rapid mid-diastolic flow into a left ventricle with reduced compliance. The auscultatory counterpart is the "ventricular knock" (see Chapter 6). When an "X" mark is placed over the left ventricular impulse, the diastolic movement is readily seen.

The precordial diastolic movement in chronic constrictive pericarditis has been called the "diastolic heartbeat." The movement coincides with rapid early diastolic flow into the constricted ventricles (left and right) and is synchronous with the brisk Y trough in the right atrial and jugular venous pulse and the early diastolic dip in the ventricular pressure pulse (see Fig. 4–11).

Let us now turn to *right* ventricular mid-diastolic impulses. The appropriate position for the patient is supine—not the left lateral decubitus—with the thorax elevated 30 degrees. The fingertips are applied—one at a time or simultaneously (see Figs. 5–7 and 5–8)—at the left sternal edge in the fourth and fifth interspaces while the breath is held in full but comfortable expiration (adult). Subxiphoid palpation (see Fig. 5–9), especially during held inspiration (older child or adult), is sometimes even more sensitive for the detection of right ventricular mid-diastolic movement. This is so, in part, because inspiration augments right ventricular filling and atrioventricular flow. Conditions necessary for generating a mid-diastolic right ventricular impulse are analogous to those described above for a left ventricular mid-diastolic impulse. The "diastolic heartbeat" of chronic constrictive pericarditis is just as likely to be palpated over the right ventricle as over the left. Chronic severe tricuspid regurgitation, especially in the presence of reduced right ventricular compliance, is another case in point.

Presystolic Movements of the Ventricles. Active atrial filling of the ventricles (atrial transport) occurs in presystole (late diastole) (Fig. 5–21) but normally is not accompanied by palpable or visible movement of either the left or right ventricle. However, when the atrial contribution to ventricular filling is augmented, as in aortic stenosis or systemic hypertension in the left heart (Figs. 5–20 and 5–22A) or pulmonic stenosis or pulmonary hypertension in the right heart (Fig. 5–22B), the velocity and amplitude

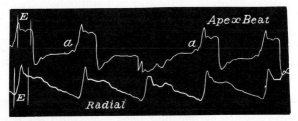

FIGURE 5–21. "Simultaneous tracings of the apex beat and of the radial pulse showing . . . the small wave (a) due to auricular systole. The third beat of the apex tracing is obliterated by the movement of inspiration" (from Mackenzie[3]).

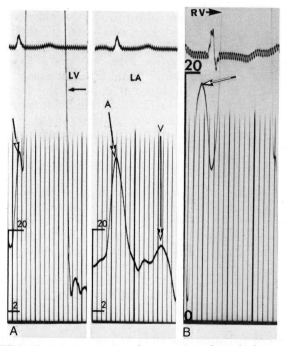

FIGURE 5–22. *A,* Severe aortic valve stenosis with marked presystolic distention *(arrow)* of the *left* ventricle (LV) in response to powerful contraction of the left atrium (LA) that generates a large A wave. The V wave is small. *B,* Primary pulmonary hypertension with marked presystolic distention *(arrow)* of the *right* ventricle (RV).

of presystolic movement reach a threshold that permits clinical detection by palpation and sometimes by observation. Mackenzie was aware of "distention of the ventricle by the auricular systole."[3]

When the *left* ventricle is under scrutiny, the patient is positioned in a partial left lateral decubitus position with the thorax elevated 30 degrees. The left ventricular impulse should be palpated with a single fingertip while the breath is held in full but comfortable expiration. The fingertip should be applied lightly, because presystolic movement (as mid-diastolic movement) is low-frequency and readily damped by firm pressure. The tactile sensation imparted to the fingertip varies from subtle, brief, and indistinct to an obvious impact immediately preceding the left ventricular systolic impulse (Fig. 5–22A). The auscultatory counterpart is the fourth heart sound (see Chapter 6); presystolic distention is often more readily palpated than the fourth sound is heard. Potain (1876) called attention to this point: "If one applies the ear to the chest, it affects the tactile sensation more perhaps than the auditory sense."[6] A subtle presystolic impulse can be reinforced (augmented) by transiently stressing the left ventricle with isometric exercise (sustained hand grip) (see Chapter 6). An X mark on the skin over the left ventricular impulse often permits ready observation of presystolic movement immediately before the major systolic impulse of the left ventricle.

Right ventricular presystolic distention is best identified with the patient in the *supine* position and the trunk either horizontal or preferably elevated 30 degrees. The fingertips are applied in the fourth and fifth left intercostal spaces during full, held expiration (see Fig. 5–7), but it may be better to palpate each interspace separately, especially in infants (see Fig. 5–8). *Subxiphoid* palpation during held *inspiration* is sometimes even more informative than left precordial palpation, because a right ventricular presystolic impulse tends to increase during inspiration.

It comes as no surprise that mid-diastolic *and* presystolic distention of either right or left ventricle may coexist (see Fig. 5–20). Identification of both of these diastolic impulses is more readily achieved when the cardiac rate is slow. A rapid rate, especially if the PR interval is long (early atrial transport), results in summation of the two ventricular filling phases, so a single, reinforced diastolic impulse results.

Movements of the Atria During Ventricular Systole. Systolic expansion of a dilated left or right atrium in patients with mitral or tricuspid regurgitation imparts distinctive movements to the chest wall. Anterior movement due to systolic expansion of the left atrium was dealt with earlier (see Fig. 5–18). In addition, a *giant* left atrium may extend well into the right hemithorax, so

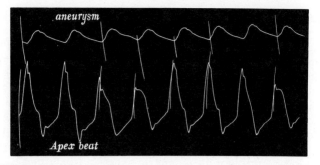

FIGURE 5–23. "Tracings from a large aneurysm pulsating in the second right intercostal space and from the apex beat" (Mackenzie[3]).

mitral regurgitation can cause late systolic movement of the lower *right* anterior chest, occasionally as far as the right anterior axillary line. When mitral regurgitation occurs in the presence of a dilated left atrial *appendage*, an impulse is palpated and often seen in the third left interspace because the appendage is border-forming at that site. Systolic expansion of the *right* atrium is sometimes palpated and seen. The right atrium normally forms the right lower cardiac border. In addition, the right lobe of the liver is just beneath the lateral and anterior rib cage. Accordingly, in the presence of chronic severe tricuspid regurgitation, the right atrium and liver enlarge appreciably, making broad contact with the anterior and lateral chest walls, which transmit the systolic pulsations. Systolic expansion of the large right atrium together with systolic movement of the large right hepatic lobe cause dramatic late systolic movement of the entire right lower chest. The right ventricle, even though volume-loaded, causes relatively less impressive anterior movement, so the chest, especially if viewed from the patient's feet, exhibits a striking rocking motion with each ventricular systole. When tricuspid *stenosis* occurs with a large, powerfully contracting right atrium, a *presystolic* impulse is sometimes transmitted to the lower right anterior chest.

Movements of the Great Arteries. The ascending aorta is normally border-forming at the right thoracic inlet but is palpable only when abnormal in size or position. An ascending aortic aneurysm (dilated aortic root in the Marfan syndrome, for example) causes a systolic impulse in the second, or first and second, right intercostal space near the sternum (Fig. 5–23). A saccular luetic aneurysm of the ascending aorta may present similarly or can burrow through the chest wall and present as a dramatic, visible pulsatile mass (Fig. 5–24). If an ascending aortic aneurysm is sufficiently cephalad (dissecting aneurysm, for instance), systolic movement may be transmitted to the right sternoclavicular joint. A systolic impulse imparted to the *left* sternoclavicular joint sometimes results

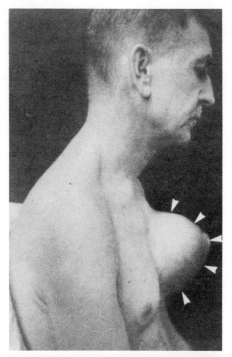

FIGURE 5–24. Saccular ascending luetic aortic aneurysm that burrowed through the chest wall as a dramatic, visible mass *(arrows)*. (From Cabot, R. C.: Physical Diagnosis. New York, William Wood and Company, 1915. Courtesy of Dr. Sherman M. Mellinkoff, UCLA Medical Center.)

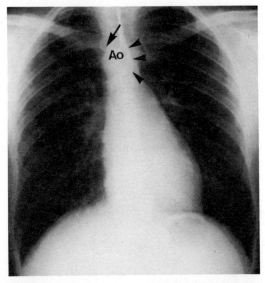

FIGURE 5–25. Radiograph of a 19-year-old male with an isolated right aortic arch (Ao) that displaces the barium-filled esophagus to the left *(arrowheads)*. The proximity of the right aortic arch to the overlying right sternoclavicular junction *(arrow)* caused a gentle systolic impulse, especially during held expiration.

from extension of the transverse portion of a dissecting aortic aneurysm. Systolic movement of the right sternoclavicular joint is a subtle sign of a right aortic arch (Fig. 5–25), particularly if the aortic root is dilated. Severe Fallot's tetralogy, especially with pulmonary atresia and dilated right aortic root, is an example. Sternoclavicular joint pulsations are rarely visible, are generally subtle, and are best sensed by relatively firm pressure with two apposed fingertips, which fix the point under examination.

Rarely, late systolic anterior movement of the sternum (and of the contiguous left parasternal area) is caused by a large, pulsatile *descending* aortic aneurysm as it phasically moves the heart forward during ventricular systole. If this sign is suspected, a *synchronous* late systolic movement should be sought in the *posterior* thorax to the left of the vertebral column.

The *pulmonary trunk* (main pulmonary artery) is normally border-forming in the second left interspace (see Fig. 5–5). To elicit an overlying systolic impulse, the patient should be examined supine, either horizontal or preferably with the thorax elevated 30 degrees. The impulse is often better seen than palpated, especially when observed during full held expiration with the site marked with an X. Detection by palpation requires a fingertip gently applied during held expiration. Mackenzie recorded systolic movement imparted by the pulmonary trunk[3] (Fig. 5–26). He wrote, " . . . through the thin chest wall the various movements of the heart could easily be observed. In the second left interspace there was a marked pulsation. The tracings of the pulsation, taken at the same time as the carotid pulse, left no doubt as to its being caused by the pulmonary artery." In thin patients, especially with decreased anteroposterior chest dimensions, a normal pulmonary trunk sometimes transmits a visible and palpable impulse to the second left interspace, especially during full held expiration. An abnormal pulmonary arterial systolic impulse occurs when the trunk is dilated (pulmonary hypertension, idiopathic dilatation), but especially when dilatation is accompanied by an increase in pulsatile excursion, as in ostium secundum atrial septal defect.

Palpable Heart Sounds. Mid-diastolic and presystolic distention of the ventricles, which represent movements

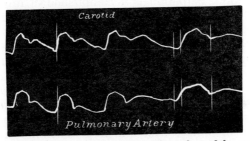

FIGURE 5–26. "Simultaneous tracings of the pulses of the carotid and pulmonary artery" (from Mackenzie[3]).

associated with low-frequency third and fourth heart sounds, have been discussed. The following remarks deal with higher-frequency sounds that are palpable because of their intensity, not because they impart movement to the chest wall. These higher-frequency sounds include loud first and second heart sounds, ejection sounds, opening snaps, and occasionally "tumor plops." Identification by palpation is analogous to the sensing of transmitted murmurs (thrills) (see below).

A prominent first heart sound (mitral component) is sometimes palpable over the left ventricular impulse in the left lateral decubitus position during held expiration in thin, slightly built subjects, especially if the PR interval is short and the cardiac rate rapid. Palpation is best accomplished by relatively firm pressure of a fingertip. In rheumatic mitral stenosis with mobile anterior leaflet, a loud first heart sound is often more readily palpable than the accompanying left ventricular impulse. The first heart sound may be loud enough to radiate to the left sternal edge and occasionally to the base. An ejection sound accompanying congenital aortic valve stenosis (see Chapter 6) is sometimes palpated, more readily so over the left ventricular impulse than in the second right interspace, and must therefore be distinguished from a loud first heart sound. A normal PR interval and a relatively slow heart rate assist in this distinction. Aortic ejection sounds that originate *within* a dilated aortic root (in contrast to origin in the valve itself) are better palpated at the right base over the site of systolic movement of the dilated aorta. Palpation is accomplished at this site by moderately firm pressure of a fingertip applied during held expiration or by firmly applying the distal metacarpals. Pulmonic ejection sounds are palpable in the second left intercostal space and are sometimes sensed only during normal expiration, diminishing or vanishing altogether during normal inspiration (see Chapter 6).

The *aortic* component of the *second heart sound* is often palpable in the second right interspace in the presence of simple systemic hypertension. The aortic closure sound is also palpable when the aortic root is dilated and the pulmonary trunk small (as in severe

Fallot's tetralogy or pulmonary atresia) or when the aortic root is anterior to the pulmonary trunk (as in complete transposition of the great arteries).

The *pulmonic component* of the second heart sound is palpated in the second left interspace in patients with pulmonary hypertension, although dilatation of the pulmonary trunk with normal pulmonary arterial pressure occasionally renders the pulmonic component palpable. In some normal children and adolescents and in thin subjects with decreased anteroposterior chest dimensions, a normal pulmonic component of the second heart sound is occasionally palpated as a gentle tap. Palpation is enhanced when a fingertip is applied between the ribs in the second left intercostal space with moderate pressure during held expiration. Pressure at the same site with the distal metacarpals is also useful. A very loud pulmonic component transmits widely to the mid and lower left sternal edge, right base, and apex, especially when the right ventricle occupies the apex.

The most common *early diastolic sound* amenable to palpation because of intensity per se is the opening snap of mitral stenosis. The sound is palpable over the left ventricular impulse, but when loud, radiates to the lower left sternal edge. A relatively rare palpable early diastolic sound—the "tumor plop" (see Chapter 6)—is generated during abrupt deceleration of a mobile, pedunculated right or left atrial myxoma as the tumor seats within the tricuspid or mitral orifice.

Palpable Murmurs—Thrills. A thrill, by definition, is a palpable murmur. The term "palpable thrill" is therefore redundant. Accordingly, a thrill should be identified as present or absent but not as palpable or impalpable.

Murmurs that reach or exceed grade IV out of VI in intensity are usually transmitted through the chest wall as thrills, but frequency composition also affects murmur transmission. Nevertheless, the presence of a thrill implies that a murmur is grade IV or more. The distal metacarpals are especially useful for the detection of thrills, although fingertips assist in precise localization. Thrills are most readily characterized according to their timing in the cardiac cycle (systolic, diastolic, or continuous), their location, their direction of radiation, and their duration. Systolic thrills at the right or left base (aortic valve stenosis, pulmonic valve stenosis) can be palpated with the patient supine at 30 to 45 degrees, or still better with the patient sitting and leaning forward during full held expiration. When the thrill is prominent and widespread, application of the entire palm of the hand is sometimes helpful in sensing the direction of radiation of the aortic stenotic thrill upward and to the right, and radiation of the pulmonic stenotic thrill upward and to the left. If the thrill is highly localized, relatively firm application of a fingertip usually suffices, but in adults, application of the metacarpals may assist.

It is useful to localize the site of maximum intensity of a left parasternal systolic thrill. Maximum intensity in the second intercostal space occurs in pulmonic *valve* stenosis, in the third intercostal space in *infundibular* pulmonic stenosis, and in the fourth or fifth intercostal space with *ventricular septal defect*. Two or three fingertips can be applied simultaneously in the second, third and fourth, or fourth, fifth and sixth interspaces, as shown in Figure 5–7. Selective, sequential lifting and reapplication of the fingertips often refines the examiner's discrimination. In infants, a single fingertip is applied to each interspace in sequence (Fig. 5–8). Most systolic thrills are better identified during expiration, but the thrill of tricuspid regurgitation is better sensed or may appear only during inspiration.

An *early diastolic left parasternal thrill* is more likely to accompany aortic regurgitation, less likely the Graham Steel murmur of high-pressure pulmonary regurgitation because the latter is usually grade III or less. The best technique for eliciting these left parasternal high-frequency early diastolic thrills is by applying the distal metacarpals or fingertips at the left sternal edge with the patient first supine at 30 to 45 degrees and then sitting and leaning forward during full held expiration. When aortic regurgitation is caused by eversion of a cusp, the frequency composition of the diastolic murmur sometimes results in transmission of a thrill more readily than would be anticipated based upon intensity alone. When the diastolic thrill of aortic regurgitation is better detected at the right sternal edge, the cause is likely to be a dilated aortic root, as in the Marfan syndrome.

Systolic and diastolic thrills over the left ventricular impulse are best assessed during held expiration with the patient in a partial left lateral decubitus position. An intense systolic thrill of mitral regurgitation commonly radiates into the axilla, sometimes to the left sternal edge, to the base, and even into the neck. Detection of the diastolic or presystolic thrill of mitral stenosis requires special care. With the patient in the left lateral decubitus position, the left ventricular impulse must first be identified, because mitral stenotic thrills are highly localized to that site. If the left ventricular impulse is inconspicuous (as it often is in this setting), palpation of the loud first heart sound assists in identifying the apex. A fingertip is then applied with pressure varying from gentle to moderate. Equivocal thrills often become more pronounced when the patient voluntarily coughs briskly, a maneuver that transiently increases the heart rate and mitral flow (see Chapter 6).

When thrills are present in systole and diastole, a distinction must be made between two separate thrills and a single continuous thrill. The continuous thrill of patent ductus arteriosus is maximal beneath the left clavicle, begins in systole, is reinforced before and after the second heart sound, and proceeds into diastole without interruption. By contrast, the "see-saw" systolic/diastolic thrills of aortic stenosis and regurgitation are maximal at the right base or mid-left sternal edge and are interrupted between the systolic and diastolic portions. More difficult and sometimes impossible to distinguish from a continuous thrill is the holosystolic thrill of ventricular septal defect or mitral regurgitation followed immediately by an early diastolic thrill of aortic regurgitation (see Chapter 6).

REFERENCES

1. Harvey, W.: An Anatomical Disquisition on the Motion of the Heart and Blood in Animals. London, 1628 (translated from the Latin by

Robert Willis, Barnes, Surrey, England, 1847). *In* Willius, F. A., and Keys, T. E.: Classics of Cardiology, Vol. 1. Malabar, Florida, Robert E. Krieger Publishing Co., 1983.

2. Laënnec, R. T. H.: Treatise on Mediate Auscultation, 1819. First American edition, Philadelphia, James Webster, 1823.

3. Mackenzie, J.: The Study of the Pulse, Arterial, Venous, and Hepatic, and of the Movements of the Heart. Edinburgh, Young J. Pentland, 1902.

4. Auenbrugger, L.: On Percussion of the Chest. Vienna, 1761 (translated by Forbes, J.: Diseases of the Chest. London, T. and G. Underwood, Fleet Street, 1824).

5. Boicourt, O. W., Nagle, R. E., and Mounsey, J. P. D.: The clinical significance of systolic retraction of the apical impulse. Br. Heart J. 27:379, 1965.

6. Potain, P. C.: Concerning the cardiac rhythm called gallop rhythm. Bull. Mem. Soc. Med. Hop. Paris 12:137, 1876. *In* Major, R. H.: Classic Descriptions of Disease. 3rd ed. Springfield, Illinois, Charles C Thomas, Publisher, 1948.

6

AUSCULTATION—THE AUDIBLE LANGUAGE OF THE HEART

With each movement of the heart, when there is the delivery of a quantity of blood from the veins to the arteries, a pulse takes place and can be heard within the chest.

DE MOTU CORDIS (1628)

The word *auscultation* is applied to the examination, made by means of the ear, of the different sounds which the circulation of the air, the reverberation of the voice, or the beatings of the heart, produce in the cavity of the chest.

Auscultation may be mediate or immediate. The application of the naked ear to the different points of the chest, is called *immediate auscultation*. It is not only inconvenient and disagreeable in many cases both to the patient and physician; but it is besides, far from giving the satisfactory results which it would seem to promise. . . . These numerous inconveniences prevent us from having recourse to this method as often as we would wish; but it has now been superseded by another. I mean the use of the stethoscope, an instrument as simple in its construction, as it is easy in its application, and which M. Laënnec has shown to be so fruitful in results, so advantageous, I will even say indispensable, in the practice of medicine.[1]

This testimony to the indispensability of mediate auscultation was written by William Stokes at age 21 years in *An Introduction to the Use of the Stethoscope* (1825). But Ernest Craige now asks whether auscultation should be rehabilitated.[2] "Should it be reserved for the occupational therapy of a dwindling coterie of antiquarians, or should it be promoted more vigorously as a viable part of our diagnostic armamentarium?'' Contemporary clinicians still carry their stethoscopes with them, but more often than not as a symbolic gesture to a distinguished past. Auscultation *should* be rehabilitated, but "to decipher the auscultatory language of diseases of the heart easily and accurately is an affair requiring labor and use and docility."[3]

The modern era of cardiac auscultation began in 1816 with Rene Theophile Hyacinthe Laënnec. A painting in the Necker Hospital in Paris shows Laënnec sitting at the bedside with his ear applied to a patient's thorax, but he considered direct or immediate auscultation, "as inconvenient for the physician as for the patient, distaste alone renders it almost impractical in the hospital; it cannot even be proposed to most women and in most of them the volume of the breast is a physical obstacle to its use."[4] The alternative was Laënnec's stethoscope. Here is his original description:

> In 1816, I was consulted by a young woman laboring under general symptoms of diseased heart, and in whose case percussion and the application of the hand were of little avail on account of the great degree of fatness. The other method just mentioned being rendered inadmissable by age and sex of the patient, I happened to recollect a simple and well-known fact of acoustics, and fancied at the same time, that it might be turned to some use on the present occasion. The fact I allude to is the augmented impression of sound when conveyed through certain solid bodies, as when we hear the scratch of a pin at one end of a piece of wood, on applying our ear to the other. Immediately, on this suggestion, I rolled a quire of paper into a sort of cylinder and applied one end of it to the region of the heart and the other to my ear, and was not a little surprised and pleased, to find that I could thereby perceive the action of the heart in a manner much more clear and distinct than I had ever been able to do by the immediate application of the ear. From this moment, I imagined that the circumstance might furnish means for enabling us to ascertain the character, not only of the action of the heart, but of every species of sound produced by the motion of all the thoracic viscera.

THE HEART SOUNDS

Heart sounds are relatively brief, discrete auditory vibrations of varying intensity (loudness), frequency (pitch),

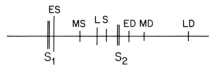

FIGURE 6–1. Heart sounds within the auditory framework established by the first heart sound (S_1) and the second heart sound (S_2). The additional heart sounds are designated descriptively as early systolic (ES), midsystolic (MS), late systolic (LS), early diastolic (ED), mid-diastolic (MD), and late diastolic (LD) or presystolic.

and quality (timbre). The first heart sound identifies the onset of ventricular systole and the second heart sound the onset of diastole. These two auditory events establish an auscultatory framework within which other heart sounds or murmurs can be placed (Fig. 6–1).

The basic heart sounds are the first, second, third, and fourth sounds (Fig. 6–2). Each can be normal or abnormal. Other heart sounds are, more often than not, abnormal, whereas still others are iatrogenic (prosthetic valve sounds, for example). The heart sounds are initially assigned simple descriptive terms that identify *where* in the cardiac cycle a given sound is occurring. Accordingly, heart sounds within the framework established by the first and second sounds are designated as "early systolic, midsystolic, late systolic" and "early diastolic, mid-diastolic, and late diastolic (presystolic)" (Fig. 6–1 and Table 6–1). The next step is to draw conclusions regarding what a sound so identified might represent (Tables 6–2 and 6–

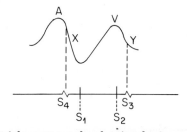

FIGURE 6–2. Atrial pressure pulse showing the A wave and X descent and the V wave and Y descent. The fourth heart sound (S_4) coincides with the atrial contraction phase of ventricular filling. The third heart sound (S_3) coincides with the Y descent (the phase of rapid ventricular filling). S_1 = first heart sound; S_2 = second heart sound.

TABLE 6–1. Heart Sounds Within the Framework of the First and Second Sounds: Descriptive Terminology

Systolic sounds	Diastolic sounds
Early systolic	Early diastolic
Midsystolic	Mid-diastolic
Late systolic	Late diastolic

TABLE 6–2. Systolic Sounds

Early Systolic	**Mid/Late Systolic**
Ejection sounds (aortic/pulmonic)	Mitral clicks
Aortic prosthetic valve sounds	"Remnants" of pericardial rubs

3). An *early systolic* sound might be an ejection sound (aortic or pulmonic) or an aortic prosthetic sound. *Mid/late* systolic sounds are typified by the click(s) of mitral valve prolapse but occasionally are "remnants" of pericardial rubs. *Early diastolic* sounds are represented by opening snaps (usually mitral), early third heart sounds (the early diastolic sound of constrictive pericarditis, or the "ventricular knock" of mitral regurgitation), the opening of a rigid mitral prosthesis, or the abrupt seating of a pedunculated mobile atrial myxoma ("tumor plop"). *Mid-diastolic* sounds are generally third heart sounds or occasionally summation sounds (synchronous occurrence of third and fourth heart sounds). *Late diastolic* or *presystolic* sounds are almost always fourth heart sounds, rarely pacemaker sounds.

TABLE 6–3. Diastolic Sounds

Early Diastolic
  Opening sounds (snaps)
  Early S_3 (early diastolic sound of constrictive pericarditis, "ventricular knock" of mitral regurgitation)
  Mitral prosthetic valve sound
  "Tumor plop"
Mid-Diastolic
  Third heart sound
  Summation sound $(S_3 + S_4)$
Late Diastolic (Presystolic)
  Fourth heart sound
  Pacemaker sound

Technique and Principles. The topographic areas for cardiac auscultation are best designated by unambiguous descriptive terms—the cardiac apex, the left and right sternal borders interspace by interspace, and subxiphoid. These topographic terms are analogous to those recommended for palpation (see Chapter 5). Terms such as "mitral area," "tricuspid area," "pulmonic area," and "aortic area" are avoided, because they assume situs solitus without ventricular inversion and with normally related great arteries. Percussion should precede auscultation in order to establish visceral and cardiac situs, so that auscultation can be conducted with topographic confidence. I recommend that auscultation then begin at the cardiac apex and contiguous lower left sternal edge (inflow), proceeding interspace by interspace up the left sternal edge to the left base and then to the right base (outflow). This topographic sequence permits the examiner to think physiologically by using an order that conforms to the direction of blood flow—inflow/outflow. It has also been recommended that auscultation begin at the base where the first and second heart sounds are more readily identified. With few exceptions, however, timing of the first heart sound can be established by simultaneous palpation of the carotid artery with the thumb of the free left hand (Fig. 6–3). In addition to the routine sites described above, the stethoscope should be applied regularly to certain nonprecordial thoracic areas, especially the axillae, the back, and the anterior chest on the opposite side.

The information derived from auscultation benefits from knowledge of cardiac situs (see above) and from identification of the movements of the ventricles. I begin by applying the stethoscope to the cardiac apex with the patient in the left lateral decubitus position (Fig. 6–3), especially when the left ventricle occupies the apex. Once the first heart sound is identified (simultaneous carotid palpation) (Fig. 6–3), auscultation then proceeds by systematic, methodical, sequential attention to early, mid, and late systole, the second heart sound, then early, mid, and late diastole (presystole), returning to the first heart sound (see Fig. 6–1). It is intuitive that auscultation

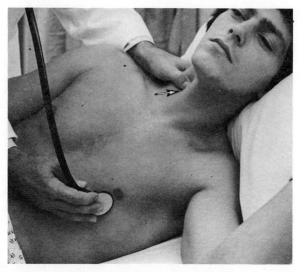

FIGURE 6–3. The bell of the stethoscope is applied to the cardiac apex while the patient lies in a partial left lateral decubitus position. The thumb of the examiner's free left hand is used to palpate the carotid artery for timing purposes *(arrow)*.

should be conducted systematically as just described. The examiner's attention and analysis should not be distracted by single dramatic auscultatory signs such as a loud murmur; otherwise less obvious although important signs are likely to be missed.

Assessment of pitch or frequency within a range of low to moderately high can be achieved by variable pressure with the stethoscopic bell, whereas for high frequencies, the diaphragm is better. It is therefore practical to begin by using the stethoscopic bell with varying pressure at the apex and lower left sternal edge, changing to the diaphragm when the base is reached. Low frequencies are best heard by applying the bell just lightly enough to establish a skin seal. High-frequency events are best elicited by firm pressure of the diaphragm.

During the course of auscultation, respiratory patterns, position, and physical interventions are important. Each of these points will be dealt with in the subsequent discussions.

The First Heart Sound. The major initial component of the first heart sound is most prominent at the cardiac apex when the apex is occupied by the left ventricle. A second component may be heard at the lower left sternal edge, less commonly at the apex, and seldom at the base. The weight of evidence indicates that the first major component is associated with closure of the mitral valve and coincides with abrupt arrest of leaflet motion when the cusps—especially the larger and more mobile anterior cusp—reach their fully closed position (maximal excursion into the left atrium). The origin of the second major component of the first heart sound is assigned to closure of the tricuspid valve based upon an analogous line of reasoning. Ejection into the great arteries (aortic root or pulmonary trunk) usually produces no audible sound in the normal heart, although phonocardiograms may record a low-amplitude sound following the mitral and tricuspid components and coinciding with the maximal opening excursions of the aortic cusps.

In addition to the presence and degree of splitting, the first heart sound should be characterized according to its quality and intensity. Because the two major audible components are believed to originate in the closing movements of the atrioventricular valves, the quality of the two components (pitch) is similar and best appreciated with relatively firm pressure of the stethoscopic bell or with the diaphragm. When the first heart sound is audibly split, its first component is normally the louder. The softer second component is confined to the apex and lower left sternal edge. Only the louder first component is normally heard at the base. The intensity of the first heart sound, particularly its first major audible component, depends chiefly upon the position of the bellies of the mitral leaflets, especially the anterior leaflet, at the time the left ventricle begins to contract and less upon the rate of left ventricular contraction. Accordingly, the first heart sound—especially its first component—is loudest when the beginning of left ventricular systole finds the mitral leaflets maximally recessed into the ventricular cavity as in the presence of a short PR interval, a rapid heart rate, short cycle lengths in atrial fibrillation, and mitral stenosis with a mobile anterior leaflet.

Early Systolic Sounds. An ejection sound (aortic or pulmonic) is the most common early systolic sound (see Fig. 6–1). The ejection sound coincides with the timing of the excursion of the relevant semilunar valve at its fully opened position, as in congenital aortic valve stenosis, bicuspid aortic valve, or dilated aortic root in the left heart, or pulmonic valve stenosis or dilated pulmonary trunk in the right heart. Ejection sounds are relatively high frequency, hence the designation "ejection click." I prefer the term "ejection sound" and reserve the term "click" for mid to late systolic sounds of mitral origin (see below) in order to avoid the rather awkward term "nonejection click" for the latter.

Ejection sounds, because of their frequency composition, should be assessed with the stethoscopic diaphragm or with firm pressure of the bell. The ejection sound of congenital aortic valve stenosis or bicuspid aortic valve is characteristically heard best over the left ventricular impulse (Fig. 6–4A) rather than at the right base. The presence of this ejection sound implies that the stenotic

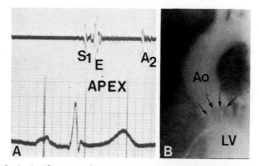

FIGURE 6–4. *A,* Phonocardiogram over the left ventricular impulse in a patient with mild congenital aortic valve stenosis. The aortic ejection sound (E) is louder than the first heart sound (S₁). A₂ = aortic component of the second heart sound. *B,* Left ventriculogram (LV) in another patient with congenital aortic valve stenosis. The cephalad systolic doming of the stenotic valve *(arrows)* produces the aortic ejection sound.

aortic valve is mobile, because the sound is caused by abrupt cephalad doming (Fig. 6–4B). The ejection sound of congenital pulmonic valve stenosis is typically confined to the second left intercostal space and is caused by abrupt cephalad doming of the mobile pulmonic stenotic valve (Fig. 6–5B). The pulmonic ejection sound often distinctively and selectively decreases in intensity during normal inspiration (Fig. 6–5A). This is so because the inspiratory increase in right atrial contractile force is transmitted into the right ventricle and to the undersurface of the mobile stenotic valve, moving its cusps upward *before* the onset of right ventricular contraction. The result is a diminished cephalad excursion of the valve during inspiration, accounting for the inspiratory decrease in intensity of the ejection sound.

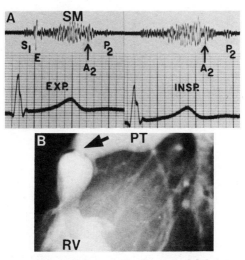

FIGURE 6–5. *A,* Phonocardiogram in the second left interspace of a patient with congenital pulmonic valve stenosis. The ejection sound (E) is obvious during expiration (EXP.) but disappears entirely during casual inspiration (INSP.). The pulmonic component of the second heart sound (P_2) is delayed. SM = systolic murmur; S_1 = first heart sound. *B,* Right ventriculogram (RV) in another patient with pulmonic valve stenosis. The cephalad systolic doming of the stenotic valve *(arrow)* produces the pulmonic ejection sound. There is poststenotic dilatation of the pulmonary trunk (PT).

The source of an ejection sound in *dilatation* of the aortic root or pulmonary trunk may also be valvular (the timing is appropriate). Origin in the wall of the dilated great artery—sudden early systolic distention—has not been excluded.

An aortic ejection sound following a first heart sound at the cardiac apex (see Fig. 6–4A) must be distinguished from a split first heart sound. The quality of the two sounds may be similar if not identical, and both sounds are well heard with the diaphragm of the stethoscope or firm pressure of the bell. However, a split first heart sound is likely to occur with a louder *first* (mitral) component, whereas a first heart sound followed by an aortic ejection sound is likely to be represented by a louder *second* component, as shown in Figure 6–4A.

An early systolic sound accompanies a ball-in-cage aortic prosthesis (especially the Starr-Edwards valve), less so with a tilting disc (such as the Bjork-Shiley valve), and not at all with a tissue prosthesis. A ball-in-cage valve sometimes produces a trill of early systolic sounds as the poppet moves upward during left ventricular systole.

Mid to Late Systolic Sounds. The most common mid to late systolic sound(s) are the clicks associated with mitral valve prolapse (Fig. 6–6). The term "click" is appropriate because these sounds are relatively high frequency and accordingly are best heard with the diaphragm of the stethoscope or firm pressure of the bell. The clicks coincide with the maximal excursion of the prolapsed leaflet(s) into the left atrium and are therefore ascribed to abrupt tensing of the redundant leaflet(s) and elongated chordae tendineae. Variability epitomizes systolic click(s), which from time to time may be present, absent, single, or multiple (Fig. 6–6) or may be replaced by a cluster of discrete late systolic "crackles." Physical interventions that *reduce* left ventricular volume, such as the Valsalva maneuver, or a change in position from supine to sitting to standing (Fig. 6–7) causes the click(s) to become earlier. Conversely, physical maneuvers that *increase* left ventricular volume such as squatting (Fig. 6–7) or sustained handgrip delay the timing of the

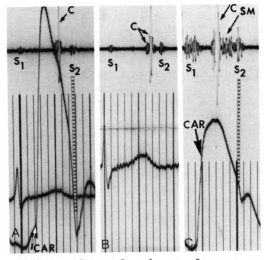

FIGURE 6–6. Phonocardiogram from the apex of a young woman with mitral valve prolapse. The tracings were recorded at different times and show *(A)* a single loud late systolic click, *(B)* a loud click still later in systole preceded by a softer click, and *(C)* a loud midsystolic click followed by a late systolic murmur. S_1 = first heart sound; S_2 = second heart sound; CAR = indirect carotid pulse; C = click.

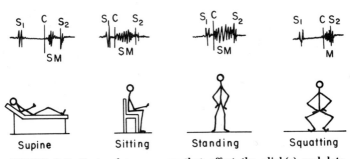

FIGURE 6–7. Postural maneuvers that affect the click(s) and late systolic murmur of mitral valve prolapse. A change from supine to sitting or standing causes the click to become earlier and the murmur longer although softer. Conversely, squatting delays the timing of the click, and the murmur gets shorter but louder. (From Circulation 54:3, 1976, with permission.)

click(s). The best way to detect mobility of the click(s) is to examine the patient during the change from squatting to prompt standing.[5]

Carl Potain, in 1894, described "small, sharp clicking sounds, well localized and such that one can scarcely attribute them to anything except the tensing of a pericardial adhesion."[6] On rare occasions, a pericardial friction rub leaves in its wake mid to late systolic sounds—remnants of rubs—that persist for varying periods of time after disappearance of the systolic phase of the rub.

The Second Heart Sound. Leatham called the second heart sound the "key to auscultation of the heart."[7] The second heart sound has two components, the first designated "aortic" and the second "pulmonic." The second sound normally splits into its two components during inspiration and is single during expiration, a respiratory variation described by Potain in 1866.[8] Splitting of the second heart sound is most readily identified in the second left intercostal space, because the softer pulmonic component is normally confined to that site, whereas the louder aortic component is heard at the base, sternal edge, and apex. "A_2" and "P_2" are appropriate terms provided that they apply to the *aortic* and *pulmonic* components as described and not to a single second heart sound in the "aortic" or "pulmonic" area.

Inspiratory splitting of the second heart sound is due chiefly to a delay in the pulmonic component, less to earlier timing of the aortic component (Fig. 6–8). The

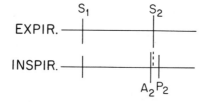

FIGURE 6–8. Normal splitting of the second heart sound. During inspiration, the second sound (S_2) splits into aortic (A_2) and pulmonic (P_2) components. The splitting is due principally to inspiratory delay in the pulmonic component (P_2).

aortic and pulmonic components of the second heart sound coincide with the aortic and pulmonary arterial dicrotic incisuras. During inspiration, the pulmonary arterial dicrotic incisura moves away from the descending limb of the right ventricular pressure pulse because of an inspiratory increase in capacitance of the pulmonary vascular bed, delaying the pulmonic component of the second heart sound (Fig. 6–8). Expiration has the opposite effect. The earlier inspiratory timing of the aortic component of the second sound is attributed to a transient reduction in left ventricular volume coupled with unchanging impedance (capacitance) in the systemic vascular bed. Accordingly, normal respiratory variations in the timing of the second heart sound are ascribed principally to the variations in impedance characteristics (capacitance) of the pulmonary vascular bed, not to an inspiratory increase in right ventricular volume as originally believed. When the increased capacitance of the normal pulmonary bed is lost because of a rise in vascular resistance, inspiratory splitting of the second sound narrows and, if present at all, reflects an increase in right ventricular ejection time and/or earlier timing of the aortic component.

Auscultatory assessment of splitting of the second heart sound is generally assessed with the patient supine or with the thorax elevated 30 to 40 degrees, but re-examination in the sitting position is sometimes useful (see below). The frequency composition of the two components of the second sound dictates use of the stethoscopic diaphragm or relatively firm pressure of the bell applied to the second left intercostal space during normal respiration. It is often helpful to instruct cooperative older children and adults regarding the rate and depth of respiration. This is accomplished by telling the patient to "breathe in" and "breathe out." The duration and depth are automatically established by the interval between the instruction to "breathe in" and the next instruction to "breathe out." In infants, the technique for assessing splitting of the second heart sound differs. The rapid, nonrhythmic breathing and the rapid heart rate conspire to prevent matching the splitting of the second heart sound with a given phase of respiration. I therefore ignore the respiratory cycle and concentrate on the second heart sound itself. If the examiner can establish with confidence that the second heart sound is at times single, and at other times clearly split, it is safe to assume that the *sequence* of semilunar valve closure is normal (aortic followed by pulmonic), because reversed or paradoxical splitting (see below) is rarely, if ever, heard in infants.

Abnormal splitting of the second heart sound falls into three general categories: (1) persistently single, (2) persistently split (fixed or nonfixed), or (3) paradoxically split (reversed). When the second sound remains single throughout the respiratory cycle, either one component is absent or the two components remain synchronous. The most common cause of a single second heart sound is simple inaudibility of the *pulmonic* component in older adults with increased anteroposterior chest dimensions (emphysema). In congenital heart disease, a single second heart sound due to absence of the pulmonic component is a feature of pulmonary atresia, severe pulmonic valve stenosis, or transposition of the great arteries (pulmonic component inaudible because of the posterior position of the pulmonary trunk). A single second heart sound due to simultaneous occurrence of its two components is a feature of Eisenmenger's complex, in which the close if not identical pulmonary and systemic vascular resistances result in aortic and pulmonary arterial dicrotic incisuras that are virtually identical in timing. A single second heart sound due to inaudibility of the aortic component occurs when the aortic valve is immobile (severe calcific aortic stenosis) or atretic (aortic atresia).

Both components of the second heart sound are sometimes absent at *all* precordial sites. This is so in older adults in whom the aortic component is absent because of severe calcific aortic stenosis and the pulmonic component is inaudible because of a large anteroposterior chest dimension.

A single semilunar valve does not necessarily generate what is perceived on auscultation as a single second heart sound. Truncus arteriosus with a quadricuspid valve is a case in point, generating what occasionally sounds like "splitting" but is due instead to asynchronous closure of multiple unequal cusps. In systemic or pulmonary hypertension (see below), a single, loud second heart sound may be sufficiently prolonged and slurred (reduplicated) to encourage the mistaken diagnosis of splitting.

Persistent splitting of the second heart sound means that the two components remain audible during both inspiration and expiration. Persistent splitting may be due to a delay in the pulmonic component, as in simple complete right bundle branch block, or to early timing of the aortic component that is occasionally present in mitral regurgitation. Appropriate inspiratory and expiratory directional changes in the interval of the split (greater with inspiration, less with expiration) identify *persistent* but not fixed splitting. This is typical of uncomplicated complete right bundle branch block, for example. Persistent splitting sometimes occurs transiently in healthy children or young adults who are examined supine, especially during shallow breathing. Re-examination in the sitting position prevents error. This simple postural maneuver generally permits a clearer impression of the normal respiratory behavior of the second heart sound, especially expiratory synchrony.

Fixed splitting of the second heart sound means that the interval between the persistently split aortic and pulmonic components remains unchanged during respiration. Fixed splitting is an auscultatory hallmark of uncomplicated ostium secundum atrial septal defect. The aortic and pulmonic components are widely separated during expiration and exhibit little or no change in the degree of splitting with inspiration or the Valsalva maneuver (see below). Wide splitting is caused by a delay in the pulmonic component because the excessive increase in pulmonary vascular capacitance delays the interval between the descending limbs of the pulmonary arterial and right ventricular pressure pulses (the "hangout" interval) and accordingly delays the pulmonic incisura and the pulmonic component of the second heart sound. Because the capacitance (impedance) of the pulmonary bed is appreciably increased, there is little or no additional increase during inspiration and little or no inspiratory delay in the pulmonic component of the second sound. The result is a fixed interval between the two widely split components. In addition, phasic changes in systemic venous return during respiration in atrial septal defect are associated with reciprocal changes in the volume of the left-to-right shunt, minimizing respiratory variations in right ventricular filling.

Paradoxic splitting of the second heart sound refers to a reversed sequence of semilunar valve closure, the pulmonic component (P_2) preceding the aortic component (A_2). The most common cause is complete left bundle branch block or a right ventricular pacemaker, both of which result in initial activation of the right side of the ventricular septum, resulting in delayed activation of the left ventricle due to transseptal (right-to-left) depolarization. Paradoxic splitting is recognized on auscultation by a second sound that separates during *expiration* and becomes single (synchronous) during *inspiration*. Inspiratory synchrony is achieved because the two components fuse due to a delay in the pulmonic component, less to earlier timing of the aortic component.

Assessment of the relative *loudness* or *intensity* of the two components of the second heart sound requires comparison of both components heard simultaneously at the same site. The relative softness of the *normal* pulmonic component is responsible for its localization in the second left interspace, whereas the relative loudness of the normal aortic component accounts for its audibility at all precordial sites. It should be restated that "A_2" properly refers to the *aortic* component and "P_2" to the *pulmonic* component, so that the term "A_2 greater than P_2" or vice versa correctly applies only when both components of the second heart sound are heard simultaneously at the same precordial site. "A_2" and "P_2" do *not* refer to a comparison of the summated second heart sound at the right and left bases. Similarly, P_2 is by definition one sound—the pulmonic component—so the expression "split P_2" is a misnomer.

An increase in intensity of the *aortic* component of the second heart sound commonly occurs in systemic hypertension. The aortic component also increases in loudness when the aorta is closer to the anterior chest wall due to aortic root dilatation or transposition of the great arteries (aorta in front of the pulmonary trunk) or when an anterior pulmonary trunk is small or absent as in pulmonary atresia.

A loud *pulmonic* component of the second heart sound is a feature of pulmonary hypertension, and the loudness is enhanced by dilatation of the hypertensive pulmonary trunk. Graham Steell, in describing the auscultatory signs of pulmonary hypertension, remarked that ". . . extreme accentuation of the pulmonary second sound is always present, the closure of the pulmonary semilunar valves being generally perceptible to the hand placed over the pulmonary area, as a sharp thud."[9] An accentuated pulmonic component of the second sound can be transmitted to the mid or lower left sternal edge and, when very loud, throughout the precordium to the apex and right base. A loud pulmonic component in the second left interspace may prevent identification of a closely preceding aortic component. In this eventuality, auscultation at other precordial sites often identifies the transmitted but attenuated pulmonic component and allows detection of splitting. A moderate increase in loudness of the pulmonic component of the second heart sound sometimes occurs in the absence of pulmonary hypertension when the pulmonary trunk is dilated, as in idiopathic dilatation or ostium secundum atrial septal defect, or with a decrease in anteroposterior chest dimensions (loss of thoracic kyphosis).

Early Diastolic Sounds. The best known early diastolic sound is the opening snap (OS) of rheumatic mitral stenosis (Fig. 6–9 and Table 6–3). The presence of an opening snap indicates that the mitral valve is mobile, at least its longer anterior leaflet, which is the source of the snap. The opening snap of mitral stenosis is high-pitched and best detected with the stethoscopic diaphragm or firm pressure of the bell at the lower left sternal edge (Fig. 6–9). The snap is less well heard at the apex, even when the left ventricle occupies the apex. A loud opening snap that radiates to the left base invites a mistaken diagnosis of wide splitting of the second heart sound.

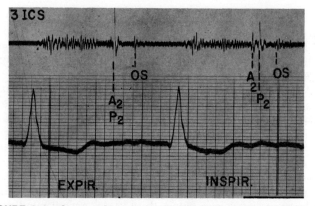

FIGURE 6–9. Phonocardiogram in the third left intercostal space (3 ICS) of a patient with rheumatic mitral stenosis. During expiration (EXPIR.), the aortic (A_2) and pulmonic (P_2) components of the second heart sound are synchronous, followed by an opening snap (OS). During inspiration (INSPIR.) three sounds are recorded—the aortic (A_2) and pulmonic (P_2) components of the split second heart sound, followed by the opening snap (OS). The A_2–OS interval is shorter in the first beat and longer in the second (variation with cycle length in atrial fibrillation).

Careful auscultation avoids this error by detecting *two* sounds during expiration (synchronous aortic and pulmonic components followed by the opening snap), but *three* sounds during inspiration (aortic component and pulmonic component followed by the opening snap) (Fig. 6–9).

The opening snap of *tricuspid* stenosis is difficult to verify by auscultation, because mitral stenosis with its snap almost invariably coexists unless the stenotic mitral valve is calcific and immobile. The snap then becomes tricuspid by exclusion. Experience enables relatively accurate prediction of the interval between the aortic component of the second heart sound and the mitral opening snap. A short interval generally means high left atrial pressure, implying significant mitral stenosis. The converse is not necessarily the case, however, because in older subjects or in the presence of systemic hypertension, tight mitral stenosis can occur with a relatively long A_2–OS interval. This is so because left ventricular systolic pressure takes longer to descend below left atrial pressure (high left ventricular systolic pressure in systemic hypertension, abnormally prolonged rate of fall of the left ventricular pressure pulse in older adults). The A_2–OS interval varies inversely with cycle length in mitral stenosis with atrial fibrillation, because (all else being equal) the higher the left atrial pressure (short cycle length), the earlier the stenotic mitral valve opens, and vice versa (Fig. 6–9).

Early diastolic sounds are features of chronic constrictive pericarditis. Dominic Corrigan, in a presentation before the Pathological Society of Dublin in December, 1842, commented on a patient with "a very loud bruit de frappement."[10] In French, *frapper* means "to knock," implying that the "bruit de frappement" was a "knocking sound" in Corrigan's patient with chronic pericarditis. The term "knock" has also been applied to an early diastolic sound in pure severe mitral regurgitation with reduced left ventricular diastolic distensibility. Corrigan's "pericardial knock" and the "ventricular knock" of mitral regurgitation are rapid filling sounds that are early and loud because a high-pressure atrium decompresses rapidly across an unobstructed atrioventricular valve into a recipient ventricle whose compliance is impaired.

An early diastolic sound in pure severe mitral regurgitation occasionally originates from a mobile anterior leaflet that opens rapidly because of the high left atrial V wave and collapsing Y descent. It is difficult, if not impossible, confidently to distinguish this "opening snap" from the "ventricular knock" of pure mitral regurgitation. The two sounds may coexist.

Early diastolic sounds are sometimes caused by atrial myxomas. The essential requirement for the generation of these sounds—"tumor plops"—is a mobile myxoma attached to the atrial septum by a long stalk. The "plop" is believed to result from abrupt diastolic seating of the mobile mass within its right or left atrioventricular orifice.

An early diastolic sound is generated by the opening movement of a rigid mitral prosthesis. The sound is especially prominent with a ball-in-cage prosthesis (Starr-

Edwards), less prominent with a tilting disc prosthesis (Bjork-Shiley), and absent with tissue valves.

Mid-diastolic and Late Diastolic (Presystolic) Sounds. In sinus rhythm, each ventricle receives blood during two diastolic filling phases (see Fig. 6–2). The first of these phases occurs when ventricular pressure drops sufficiently to allow an atrioventricular valve to open; blood then flows from atrium into ventricle. Flow coincides with the Y descent of the atrial pressure pulse (see Fig. 6–2) and is designated the rapid filling phase of ventricular diastole, accounting for about 80 per cent of normal filling. This phase is not a passive event in which inflow merely expands the recipient ventricle, but instead, ventricular relaxation is a complex, active, energy-dependent process. The sound generated during the rapid filling phase is called the third heart sound (see Fig. 6–2). The second phase—diastasis—is variable in duration, usually permitting less than 5 per cent of ventricular filling. Atrial systole initiates the third phase of diastole and accounts for about 15 per cent of normal ventricular filling. The sound generated during the atrial filling phase is called the fourth heart sound (see Fig. 6–2). The third and the fourth heart sounds both occur *within* the recipient ventricle as that chamber receives blood. Potain attributed the third heart sound to sudden cessation of distention of the ventricle in early diastole, and he attributed the fourth heart sound to ". . . the abruptness with which the dilatation of the ventricle takes place during the presystolic period, a period which corresponds to the contraction of the auricle."[11]

The presence of third and fourth heart sounds may produce a cadence called "gallop rhythm." The term is a *pathologic* designation that is inappropriate unless the causative sound, be it a third sound or fourth heart sound, is *abnormal*. Potain wrote his classic description of "cardiac rhythm called gallop rhythm" in 1876.[11] The following is the account of gallop rhythm caused by a fourth heart sound:

The formation of this rhythm of which I wish to speak, is as follows. We distinguish here three sounds, namely: the two normal sounds and an additional sound. The normal sounds show most frequently their normal characteristics, without any modification. The first especially maintains its normal relationship to the apex heart and to the arterial phase. As to the abnormal sound, it is placed immediately before it, preceding it sometimes by a very short time; always notably larger, however, than that which separates the two parts of a reduplicated sound. . . .

Gallop rhythm caused by the addition of a third *or* fourth heart sound is a *triple* rhythm (Fig. 6–10). The presence of both third *and* fourth heart sounds produce a *quadruple* rhythm (Fig. 6–10). When diastole is short or the PR interval long, the third and fourth heart sounds summate to form a summation sound or a summation gallop rhythm (Fig. 6–10).

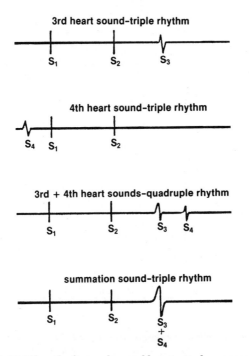

3rd heart sound–triple rhythm

S_1 S_2 S_3

4th heart sound–triple rhythm

S_4 S_1 S_2

3rd + 4th heart sounds–quadruple rhythm

S_1 S_2 S_3 S_4

summation sound–triple rhythm

S_1 S_2 S_3
                          $+$
                          S_4

FIGURE 6–10. When the first and second heart sounds are accompanied by a third (S_3) and/or a fourth heart sound (S_4), the cadence of a triple or quadruple rhythm is produced. S_3 and S_4 sometimes summate (lower tracing).

The presence of these individual sounds is much more important than the rhythm or cadence they create. When third or fourth heart sounds coexist with other sounds and/or murmurs (Fig. 6–11), the "gallop" cadence is lost. It is then appropriate to use the term "abnormal third" or "abnormal fourth" heart sound rather than to say that "gallop sounds" exist without gallop rhythm.

How can one distinguish normal from abnormal third and fourth heart sounds? Generally it is by the company they keep, rather than by distinctive auscultatory properties of the sounds themselves. The abnormal filling sounds that cause gallop rhythms are not merely exaggerations of normal third and fourth heart sounds at relatively rapid heart rates, but instead result from the inappropriate presence of the sounds, whose intensities may, in fact, be soft rather than prominent. Children and young adults often have normal (physiologic) *third* heart sounds but do not have normal fourth heart sounds. Normal third heart sounds sometimes persist beyond age 40 years, particularly in women. After that age, especially in men, the third heart sound is likely to be abnormal. Fourth heart sounds are sometimes heard, especially after exer-

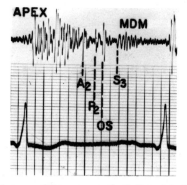

FIGURE 6–11. Phonocardiogram over the left ventricular impulse in a patient with rheumatic mitral stenosis and regurgitation. A third heart sound (S_3) introduces a short mid-diastolic murmur (MDM), but the S_3 does not result in a "gallop rhythm" because a holosystolic murmur, a split second heart sound (A_2 and P_2), an opening snap (OS), and a mid-diastolic murmur preclude the gallop cadence.

cise, in healthy older adults without clinical evidence of heart disease. Such observations have led to the belief, still debated, that these fourth heart sounds are normal. In any event, there are no significant differences in quality between normal and abnormal third and fourth heart sounds that confidently permit distinction by auscultation. Further to the point, *normal* third and fourth heart sounds are capable of creating a triple rhythm cadence, but the term "gallop rhythm" should not be applied in this context because of its pathologic connotation. The term "normal third" or "normal fourth heart sound" should be used instead.

Third and fourth heart sounds originate in either left or right ventricle. The fourth heart sound requires active atrial contribution to ventricular filling, so that fourth heart sounds disappear when coordinated contractions of the atria cease, as in atrial fibrillation. When the atria and ventricles contract independently, as in complete heart block, fourth heart sounds or summation sounds occur randomly in diastole because the relationship between the P wave and the QRS of the electrocardiogram is random. In light of the fact that third and fourth heart sounds are events of ventricular filling, obstruction of an atrioventricular valve, by impeding ventricular inflow, removes one of the prime preconditions for the generation of these sounds. In other words, the presence of a third or a fourth heart sound implies an unobstructed atrioventricular valve on its side of origin.

Third and fourth heart sounds, normal or abnormal, are relatively low-frequency events that are often soft and require special stethoscopic technique for detection. Potain called attention to this point: "The sound is dull, much more so than the normal sound. It is a shock, a perceptible elevation, it is scarcely a sound. If one applies the ear to the chest, it affects the tactile sensation, more perhaps than the auditory sense. If one attempts to hear it with a flexible stethoscope, it lacks only a little, almost always, of disappearing completely."[11] These soft, low-frequency sounds are best heard in a quiet room when the bell of the stethoscope is applied selectively over left or right ventricular impulse with just enough pressure to

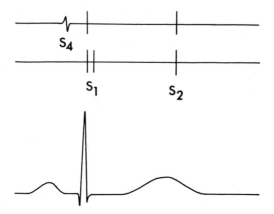

FIGURE 6–12. Illustration (upper tracing) of a low-frequency fourth heart sound (S_4) preceding a single first heart sound, and (lower tracing) a split first heart sound (S_1), the two components of which are of the same quality.

form a skin seal. Firm pressure of the bell or use of the stethoscopic diaphragm damps low-frequency vibrations and reduces audibility of third and fourth heart sounds or eliminates them altogether. These same physical properties can be used to advantage, however, in distinguishing a split first heart sound (the two components of which are preserved or enhanced by the diaphragm or pressure of the bell) from a fourth heart sound preceding a split first heart sound (the fourth heart sound is damped by pressure while the first heart sound is not) (Fig. 6–12). This distinction was addressed by Potain, who asked:

> Is the rhythm with which we are concerned nothing but a reduplication of the first heart sound? I believe this absolutely erroneous and for the following reasons. In the first place, the abnormal sound has, in no way, the timbre or usual characteristics of a valvular sound. . . . Finally (and this is the unanswerable argument that makes unnecessary all other reasons), I have heard, in certain patients, successively and in the same cardiac revolution, the "bruit de gallop" itself and a reduplication of the first heart sound. I mean that after the dull sound which constitutes the first part of the gallop rhythm, one noted clearly a doubled first sound, a reduplicated clicking of the usual type. (See Fig. 6–12).[11]

Third and fourth heart sounds originating within the

left ventricular cavity are best heard over the left ventricular impulse, especially when the impulse is brought closer to the chest wall by turning the patient into a partial left lateral decubitus position (see Fig. 6–3). *Right* ventricular third and fourth heart sounds are heard best over the *right* ventricular impulse, that is, along the lower left sternal edge or in the subxiphoid region with the patient supine. The subxiphoid site is especially appropriate in patients with emphysema.

Audibility of *third heart sounds* is improved by isotonic exercise. A few sit-ups may suffice to produce the desired increase in venous return and acceleration in heart rate that increase the rate and volume of atrioventricular flow. Venous return can be increased by simple passive raising of both legs with the patient supine and recumbent. The heart rate is also transiently increased by vigorous coughing. Left ventricular *fourth heart sounds*, especially in patients with ischemic heart disease, can be induced or augmented by increasing resistance to left ventricular discharge by sustained handgrip (isometric exercise, see below).

Right ventricular third or fourth heart sounds often respond selectively and distinctively to respiration by increasing their audibility during inspiration. Auscultation with the bell of the stethoscope in the subxiphoid region improves the sensitivity of the inspiratory maneuver by avoiding the damping effect of inspiration at the left sternal edge as the anteroposterior chest dimension increases.

When the heart rate is rapid, atrial contraction coincides with the rapid filling phase, making it impossible to determine whether an accompanying filling sound is a third heart sound, a fourth heart sound, or a summation sound (see Fig. 6–10). Carotid sinus pressure transiently slows the heart rate, so that auscultation can discriminate at which point in diastole a given sound is occurring.

Under what circumstances are abnormal third and fourth heart sounds most likely to occur?

The gallop stroke is diastolic and is due to the beginning of sudden tension in the ventricular wall as a result of the blood flow into the cavity. It is more pronounced if the wall is not distensible and the failure of distensibility may depend either on a sclerotic thickening of the heart wall (hypertrophy) or to a decrease in muscular tonicity. Since the wall, by virtue of its own elasticity, is no longer able to resist the inflow of blood, it is placed under tension precisely at the moment that this occurs.[8]

The *third* heart sound is believed to be due to sudden intrinsic limitation of longitudinal expansion of the left ventricular wall during early diastolic filling.[12] The majority of abnormal third heart sounds result from altered physical properties of the recipient ventricle and/or an increase in the rate and volume of atrioventricular flow during the rapid filling phase of the cardiac cycle.

Abnormal *fourth* heart sounds can be anticipated when augmented atrial contraction is required to produce presystolic distention of a ventricle, i.e., an increase in end-diastolic segment length, so that the ventricle can contract with greater force. Typical examples are the left ventricular hypertrophy of aortic stenosis or systemic hypertension in the left heart, or the right ventricular hypertrophy of pulmonic stenosis or pulmonary hypertension in the right heart. Fourth heart sounds are also common in ischemic heart disease and are almost universal during acute myocardial infarction, because the atrial "booster pump" is needed to assist the relatively stiff ischemic ventricle in maintaining adequate contractile force.

An interesting variation on the theme of presystolic sounds is the "pacemaker sound" (Fig. 6–13). A pacing catheter in the right ventricular apex may produce a presystolic sound that is high-pitched and clicking and therefore different in pitch from a fourth heart sound. The consensus is that the pacemaker sound is extracardiac, resulting from contraction of chest wall muscle following spread of the electrical impulse from the pacemaker.

MURMURS—SYSTOLIC, DIASTOLIC, AND CONTINUOUS

A cardiovascular murmur is a relatively prolonged series of auditory vibrations characterized according to

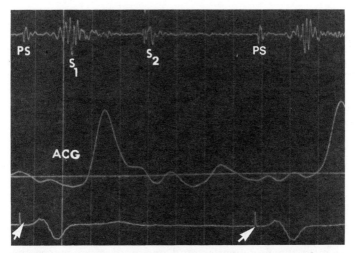

FIGURE 6–13. Phonocardiogram in the fourth left intercostal space with simultaneous apex cardiogram (ACG) and electrocardiogram in a patient with a right ventricular pacemaker. The pacemaker sound (PS) is synchronous with the pacemaker stimulus *(arrows)* shown in the electrocardiogram.

intensity (loudness), frequency (pitch), configuration (shape), quality, duration, direction of radiation, and timing in the cardiac cycle. Once these features are established by auscultation, the stage is set for diagnostic conclusions that can be drawn from a murmur of a given description. I shall emphasize the clinical assessment, physiologic mechanisms, and interpretation of murmurs, rather than the physical principles that govern their production.

The intensity or loudness of a murmur is graded from 1 to 6, based upon the original recommendations of Samuel A. Levine in 1933.[13] A grade 1 murmur is so faint that it is heard only with special effort. A grade 2 murmur is faint but readily detected; a grade 3 murmur is prominent but not loud; a grade 4 murmur is loud; and a grade 5 murmur is very loud. A grade 6 murmur is loud enough to be heard with the stethoscope just removed from contact with the chest wall. The frequency or pitch of a murmur varies from high to low. The configuration or shape of a systolic murmur is best characterized as crescendo, decrescendo, crescendo-decrescendo (diamond-shaped), plateau (even), or variable (uneven) (Fig. 6–14). The quality of a murmur is sometimes assigned descriptive terms such as harsh, rough, rumbling, scratchy, buzzing, grunting, blowing, musical, whooping, squeaking, and so forth. The duration of a murmur varies from short to long with all gradations in between. A loud murmur radiates from its site of maximal intensity, and the direction of radiation sometimes provides useful diagnostic information. The timing of a murmur within the cardiac cycle is the basis for a clinically practical classification.

There are three basic categories of murmurs—systolic, diastolic, and continuous. A *systolic* murmur begins with or after the first heart sound and ends at or before the second heart sound on its side of origin (Fig. 6–15). A *diastolic* murmur begins with or after the second heart sound and ends before the first heart sound (Fig. 6–16). A *continuous* murmur begins in systole and continues without interruption through the timing of the second heart sound into all or part of diastole (Fig. 6–17). The following descriptive classification of murmurs is based upon timing relative to the first and second heart sounds.

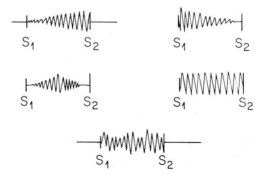

FIGURE 6–14. The five basic shapes or configurations of systolic murmurs are illustrated as crescendo, decrescendo, crescendo-decrescendo, plateau (even), and variable (uneven).

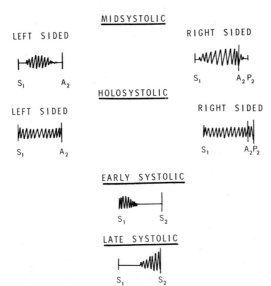

FIGURE 6–15. Systolic murmurs are descriptively classified according to their time of onset and termination as midsystolic, holosystolic, early systolic, and late systolic. Termination of the murmur must be related to the component of the second heart sound on its side of origin, that is, the aortic component (A_2) for systolic murmurs originating in the left side of the heart and the pulmonic component (P_2) for systolic murmurs originating in the right side of the heart.

Systolic Murmurs. Systolic murmurs are classified according to their time of onset and termination as midsystolic, holosystolic, early systolic, or late systolic (see Fig. 6–15). A midsystolic murmur begins after the first heart sound and ends perceptibly before the second sound. The termination of the murmur must be related to the component of the second heart sound on its side of origin (see Fig. 6–15). Midsystolic murmurs originating in the *left* heart end before the *aortic* component of the second sound; midsystolic murmurs originating in the *right* heart end before the *pulmonic* component of the second heart sound. A *holosystolic murmur* begins with the first heart sound, occupies all of systole, and ends with the second heart sound on its side of origin (see Fig. 6–15). Holosystolic murmurs originating in the *left* heart end with the

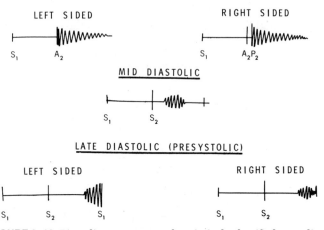

FIGURE 6–16. Diastolic murmurs are descriptively classified according to their time of *onset* as early diastolic, mid-diastolic, or late diastolic (presystolic). Diastolic murmurs originate in either the left or the right side of the heart.

aortic component of the second sound, and holosystolic murmurs originating in the *right* heart end with the pulmonic component of the second sound (see Fig. 6–15).

The term "regurgitant systolic murmur," originally applied to murmurs that occupied all of systole, has fallen into disuse, because "regurgitation" can be accompanied by midsystolic, early systolic, or late systolic murmurs. Similarly, the term "ejection systolic murmur," originally applied to midsystolic murmurs, should be discarded, because midsystolic murmurs are not necessarily due to "ejection."

MIDSYSTOLIC MURMURS. There are five settings in which midsystolic murmurs occur: (1) obstruction to ventricular outflow, (2) dilatation of the aortic root or pulmonary trunk, (3) accelerated systolic flow into the aorta or pulmonary trunk, (4) innocent midsystolic murmurs, including those due to morphologic changes in semilunar valves (generally aortic) without obstruction, and (5) some

CONTINOUS   MURMURS

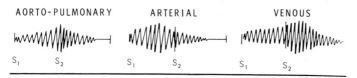

AORTO-PULMONARY   ARTERIAL   VENOUS

S₁   S₂   S₁   S₂   S₁   S₂

HOLOSYSTOLIC–EARLY   DIASTOLIC   MURMUR

SM   DM

S₁   S₂

FIGURE 6–17. Continuous murmurs begin in systole and *continue without interruption* through the second heart sound (S_2) into all or part of diastole. The continuous murmurs shown here are aortopulmonary, arterial, and venous. A holosystolic murmur (HSM) followed by a holodiastolic murmur (HDM) represents two separate murmurs, not one continuous murmur.

forms of mitral regurgitation. The physiologic mechanism of *outflow* midsystolic murmurs reflects the pattern of phasic flow across the left or right ventricular outflow tract as originally described by Leatham[14] (Fig. 6–18). Following isovolumetric contraction and the generation of the first heart sound, ventricular pressure rises to open the aortic or pulmonic valve. Ejection commences, and the murmur begins. As ejection proceeds, the murmur increases in crescendo; as ejection declines, the murmur decreases in decrescendo. The murmur ends before ventricular pressure drops below central arterial pressure, at which time the aortic and pulmonic valves close with generation of the aortic and pulmonic components of the second heart sound (Fig. 6–18).

Aortic valve stenosis is associated with a protypical midsystolic murmur which may have an early systolic peak and a short duration, a relatively late peak and a prolonged duration, or all gradations in between. Whether long or short, however, the murmur remains a symmetric diamond beginning after the first heart sound (or with an ejection sound), rising in crescendo to a systolic peak,

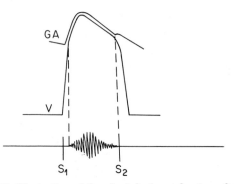

FIGURE 6–18. Illustration of the physiologic mechanism of an outflow midsystolic murmur generated by phasic flow (ejection) into the aortic root or pulmonary trunk. Ventricular (V) and great arterial (GA) pressure pulses are shown with phonocardiogram. The murmur begins after the first heart sound (S₁) when ventricular pressure exceeds the pressure in the relevant great artery. The murmur rises in crescendo to a peak as flow proceeds, then declines in decrescendo as flow diminishes, ending just before the second heart sound (S₂) as ventricular pressure falls below the pressure in the great artery.

and declining in decrescendo to end before the aortic component of the second heart sound (see Fig. 6–15) (midsystolic, left-sided). In typical aortic valve stenosis, the midsystolic murmur is loudest in the second right intercostal space with radiation upward, to the right, and into the neck because of the direction of the high-velocity jet within the aortic root. An important variation occurs in older adults in whom aortic stenosis (obstruction) or sclerosis (no obstruction, see below) is caused by fibrocalcific changes in previously normal trileaflet aortic valves. The accompanying murmur in the second right interspace is harsh, noisy, and impure, whereas the murmur over the left ventricular impulse is typically pure, often musical (Fig. 6–19). The right basal component of the murmur originates within the aortic root because of turbulence caused by the high-velocity jet (Fig. 6–19A). The pure, musical component of the murmur heard over the left ventricular impulse is ascribed to periodic high-frequency vibrations of the fibrocalcific cusps without commissural fusion (Figs. 6–19A and B). These two

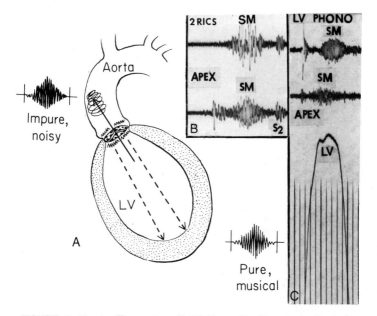

FIGURE 6–19. *A*, Illustration of "Gallavardin dissociation" of the murmurs associated with a stenotic trileaflet aortic valve in older adults. The impure, noisy midsystolic murmur at the right base originates within the aortic root because of turbulence caused by the high-velocity jet. The pure, musical midsystolic murmur at the apex results from periodic high-frequency vibrations originating in the fibrocalcific but mobile cusps and radiates selectively into the left ventricular cavity (LV). *B*, Phonocardiogram illustrating "Gallavardin dissociation." The impure, noisy midsystolic murmur (MS) is recorded in the second right intercostal space (2 RICS), while the pure, musical midsystolic murmur (MS) is recorded simultaneously at the apex. *C*, Phonocardiogram from within the left ventricular (LV) cavity records the high-frequency, musical midsystolic murmur (MS), while the microphone over the left ventricular impulse (apex) records the same murmur on the chest wall.

distinctive midsystolic murmurs—the noisy right basal and the musical apical—were described by Gallavardin in 1925,[15] and the designation "Gallavardin dissociation" is still used. The musical apical component of the midsystolic murmur is sometimes dramatically loud. William Stokes (1855) reported that such a murmur was heard at a distance of 3 feet from the chest, and that "this gentleman once observed to me that his entire body was one humming top."[16]

The apical midsystolic murmur of aortic stenosis or sclerosis requires auscultatory distinction from the apical murmur of mitral regurgitation, a difference that may be difficult or impossible to establish. In fact, the two murmurs may coexist. If the aortic component of the second heart sound is well heard at the base but inaudible at the apex, the second sound may be buried in the late systolic vibrations of an apical holosystolic murmur of mitral regurgitation. However, if the aortic valve is immobile (densely calcified), its closure sound is soft or inaudible, so the length and configuration of the apical murmur cannot be timed with the aortic component of the second heart sound. When premature ventricular contractions are followed by pauses longer than the dominant cycle length, the apical midsystolic murmur of aortic stenosis or sclerosis increases in intensity in the beat following the premature contraction, whereas the murmur of mitral regurgitation (be it midsystolic or holosystolic) remains relatively unchanged in intensity (Fig. 6–20). The same patterns hold following longer cycle lengths in atrial fibrillation. The validity of these observations assumes that aortic and mitral murmurs do not coexist at the apex.

An outflow midsystolic murmur originating in the right side of the heart is typified by the murmur of pulmonic valve stenosis (see Fig. 6–5A). The murmur begins after the first heart sound or with an ejection sound, rises in

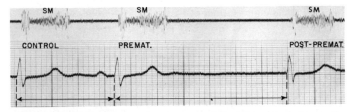

FIGURE 6–20. The effect of changes in cycle length on the holosystolic murmur (HSM) of mitral regurgitation. The intensity of the murmur changes little if at all when the control beat is compared to the post-premature beat that occurs after an increase in cycle length.

crescendo to a peak, and then declines in decrescendo to end before a delayed pulmonic component of the second heart sound (see Figs. 6–5A and 6–15) (midsystolic, right-sided). The murmur is maximal in the second left interspace with radiation upward and to the left, and, when loud, radiates to the suprasternal notch and into the base of the neck, particularly on the left side. The length and configuration of the murmur are useful signs of the degree of pulmonic stenosis. The greater the obstruction, the longer the duration of right ventricular ejection and the longer the murmur. The relative lengths of right and left ventricular ejection can be compared by relating the end of the pulmonic stenotic murmur (right-sided event) to the timing of the *aortic* component of the second heart sound (left-sided event) (see Fig. 6–5A). A soft, symmetric midsystolic murmur that ends well before the aortic component is a feature of *mild* pulmonic stenosis. A loud, asymmetric murmur that peaks in late systole (kite-shaped) and extends well beyond the aortic component of the second sound is a feature of *severe* pulmonic stenosis. There are all gradations in between (see Figs. 6–5A and 6–15).

Short, soft midsystolic murmurs can originate within a dilated aortic root or pulmonary trunk. Similar midsystolic murmurs are also generated by rapid ejection into a *normal* aortic root or pulmonary trunk as in pregnancy, fever, thyrotoxicosis, or anemia. In uncomplicated ostium secundum atrial septal defect, the pulmonic midsystolic murmur results from a combination of *rapid* ejection into a *dilated* pulmonary trunk.

Normal or *innocent* systolic murmurs are, with the exception of the systolic mammary souffle, all midsystolic (Table 6–4). The normal vibratory midsystolic murmur described by George Still (1909)[17] is short, buzzing, pure, and medium-frequency (Fig. 6–21) and is believed to originate from low-frequency periodic vibrations of normal pulmonic leaflets at their attachments. In characterizing his murmur, Still wrote:

> It is heard usually just below the level of the nipple, and about halfway between the left margin of the sternum and the vertical

TABLE 6–4. Normal Murmurs

Systolic
Vibratory systolic murmur (Still's murmur)
Pulmonic systolic murmur (pulmonary trunk)
Peripheral pulmonic systolic murmur (pulmonary branches)
Supraclavicular or brachiocephalic systolic murmur
Systolic mammary souffle
Aortic systolic murmur
Continuous
Venous hum
Continuous mammary souffle

nipple line . . . ; its characteristic feature is a twanging sound very like that made by twanging a piece of tense string. . . . Whatever may be its origin, I think it is clearly functional, that is to say, not due to any organic disease either congenital or acquired.

A second type of innocent pulmonic midsystolic murmur occurs in children, adolescents, and young adults and represents an exaggeration of normal ejection vibrations within the pulmonary trunk. The pulmonic midsystolic murmur is relatively impure and is best heard in the second left interspace, in contrast to the vibratory midsystolic murmur of Still, which is typically heard between the lower left sternal edge and apex. Normal pulmonic midsystolic murmurs are also heard in thin patients with diminished anteroposterior chest dimensions. Loss of thoracic kyphosis, for example, increases the proximity of the pulmonary trunk to the chest wall

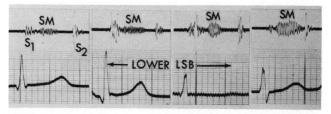

FIGURE 6–21. Four vibratory midsystolic murmurs (MS) from healthy children. These murmurs, designated "Still's murmur," are pure, medium frequency, relatively brief in duration, and maximal along the lower left sternal border (LSB). The last of the four murmurs was from a 5-year-old girl who was febrile. Following defervescence, the murmur decreased in loudness and in duration.

and increases audibility of ejection vibrations within the pulmonary trunk.

The most common form of "innocent" midsystolic murmur in older adults is designated the *"aortic sclerotic"* murmur (see above). The cause of this functionally benign murmur is fibrous or fibrocalcific thickening of the bases of otherwise normal aortic cusps as they insert into the sinuses of Valsalva. As long as the fibrosis or fibrocalcific thickening is confined to the *base* of the leaflets, the free edge moves well and there is no obstruction. The accompanying impure midsystolic murmur in the second right intercostal space results from turbulence in the aortic root, whereas the pure, high-frequency musical midsystolic murmur at the apex results from high frequency periodic vibrations of mobile aortic cusps stiffened at their attachments but without commissural fusion (see Gallavardin phenomenon described above).

It is important to underscore that some forms of *mitral regurgitation* generate midsystolic murmurs. The physiologic mechanism responsible for the midsystolic murmur of mitral regurgitation (usually associated with left ventricular wall motion abnormalities of ischemic heart disease) relates to early systolic competence of the valve and midsystolic incompetence followed by a late systolic decrease in regurgitant flow. In any event, this midsystolic murmur is not an "ejection" systolic murmur.

HOLOSYSTOLIC MURMURS (see Fig. 6–15). A holosystolic murmur begins with the first heart sound and occupies all of systole (Gr. *holos* = entire) up to the second sound on its side of origin. Such murmurs are generated by flow from a chamber or vessel whose pressure or resistance *throughout* systole is higher than the pressure or resistance in the chamber or vessel receiving the flow. Holosystolic murmurs occur in the left heart with mitral regurgitation, in the right heart with tricuspid regurgitation, between the ventricles in restrictive ventricular septal defects, and between the great arteries through an aortopulmonary window or patent ductus arteriosus when elevated pulmonary vascular resistance eliminates the diastolic shunt (see below).

The timing of holosystolic murmurs within the framework established by the first and second heart sounds reflects the physiologic and anatomic mechanisms responsible for their genesis. Figure 6–22 illustrates the mechanism of the holosystolic murmur of mitral or tricuspid regurgitation. Ventricular pressure exceeds atrial pressure at the very onset of systole, so regurgitant flow and murmur begin with the first heart sound. The murmur persists up to or slightly beyond the relevant component of the second heart sound, provided that the ventricular pressure at end-systole exceeds the atrial pressure and provided that the atrioventricular valve remains incompetent.

When the flow generating the holosystolic murmur of mitral regurgitation is directed posterolaterally within the left atrial cavity, the murmur radiates into the axilla, to the angle of the left scapula, and occasionally to the vertebral column, with bone conduction from the cervical to the lumbar spine (Fig. 6–23). When the direction of the intra-atrial jet is forward and medial against the atrial septum near the base of the aorta, the murmur radiates

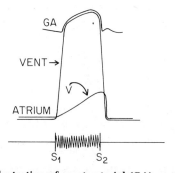

FIGURE 6–22. Illustration of great arterial (GA), ventricular (VENT), and atrial pressure pulses, with phonocardiogram, showing the physiologic mechanism of holosystolic murmurs heard in some forms of mitral and tricuspid regurgitation. Ventricular pressure exceeds atrial pressure from the onset of systole, so regurgitant flow and murmur commence with the first heart sound (S_1). The murmur persists up to or slightly beyond the second heart sound (S_2), because regurgitation persists to the end of systole (left ventricular pressure still exceeds left atrial pressure). V = atrial V wave.

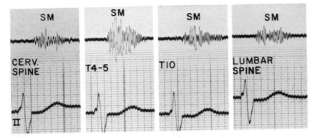

FIGURE 6–23. Radiation of the systolic murmur (SM) of pure severe mitral regurgitation to the back with bone conduction from the cervical spine to the lumbar spine.

to the left sternal edge, to the base, and even into the neck.

The murmur of tricuspid regurgitation is holosystolic when there is a substantial elevation of right ventricular systolic pressure, as schematically illustrated in Figure 6–22. A distinctive and diagnostically important feature of this murmur is an inspiratory increase in loudness—Carvallo's sign.[18] The tricuspid systolic murmur is occasionally audible *only* during inspiration. The increase in loudness occurs because the inspiratory augmentation in right ventricular volume is converted into an increase in stroke volume and in the velocity of regurgitant flow. When the right ventricle fails, this capacity is lost, so Carvallo's sign vanishes.

The murmur of an uncomplicated restrictive ventricular septal defect is holosystolic because the left ventricular systolic pressure and systemic resistance exceed right ventricular systolic pressure and pulmonary resistance from the onset to the end of systole. Holosystolic murmurs are perceived as such in patients with large aortopulmonary connections (aortopulmonary window, patent ductus arteriosus) when a rise in pulmonary vascular resistance abolishes the diastolic portion of the continuous murmur, leaving a murmur that is holosystolic or nearly so.

EARLY SYSTOLIC MURMURS (see Fig. 6–15). Early systolic murmurs begin with the first heart sound, diminish in decrescendo, and end well before the second heart sound, generally at or before midsystole. Certain types of mitral regurgitation, tricuspid regurgitation, or ventricular septal defects are examples.

Acute severe mitral regurgitation is accompanied by an early systolic murmur, or a holosystolic murmur that is decrescendo, diminishing if not ending before the second heart sound (Fig. 6–24). The physiologic mechanism responsible for this early systolic decrescendo murmur is regurgitation into a normal-sized left atrium of limited distensibility. A steep rise in left atrial V wave approaches left ventricular pressure at end-diastole; a late systolic decline in left ventricular pressure favors this tendency (Fig. 6–24). The stage is set for regurgitant flow that is maximal in early systole and minimal in late systole. The systolic murmur parallels this pattern, declining or vanishing before the second heart sound (Fig. 6–24).

An early systolic murmur is a feature of "low-pressure" tricuspid regurgitation, i.e., tricuspid regurgitation with *normal* right ventricular systolic pressure. The regurgitation accompanying tricuspid valve infective endocarditis

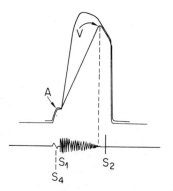

FIGURE 6–24. Ventricular and atrial pressure pulses with phonocardiogram illustrating the mechanism of the *early* systolic murmur of acute severe mitral regurgitation or low-pressure tricuspid regurgitation. The large V wave reaches ventricular pressure at end-systole *(upper curved arrow)*, so significant regurgitant flow diminishes or ceases. Accordingly, the murmur is early systolic and decrescendo, paralleling the hemodynamic pattern of regurgitant flow. S_4 = fourth heart sound.

in drug abusers is a case in point. The mechanisms responsible for the timing and configuration of early systolic murmurs of low-pressure tricuspid regurgitation are analogous to those described in the preceding paragraph and illustrated in Figure 6–24. The tall right atrial V wave reaches the level of normal right ventricular pressure in latter systole, so the regurgitation and the murmur are chiefly, if not exclusively, *early* systolic. These murmurs are medium or low frequency, because normal right ventricular systolic pressure generates a comparatively low velocity of regurgitant flow. This is in contrast to the high-frequency holosystolic murmur of tricuspid regurgitation with *elevated* right ventricular systolic pressure (see above).

Early systolic murmurs also occur in the presence of ventricular septal defects but under two widely divergent anatomic and physiologic circumstances. A soft, pure, high-frequency, early systolic murmur localized to the mid- or lower left sternal edge is typical of a very small ventricular septal defect in which the shunt is confined to early systole (Fig. 6–25). A murmur of similar timing and configuration occurs through a nonrestrictive ventric-

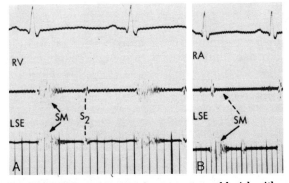

FIGURE 6–25. Phonocardiogram from a 4-year-old girl with a very small ventricular septal defect and a trivial early systolic shunt. *A*, A soft, pure, high-frequency, early systolic decrescendo murmur (SM) is recorded *within* the right ventricle (RV) and simultaneously along the lower left sternal edge (LSE). *B*, When the intracardiac microphone was withdrawn into the right atrium (RA), the murmur vanished.

ular septal defect when an elevated pulmonary vascular resistance decreases or abolishes late systolic shunting.

LATE SYSTOLIC MURMURS (see Fig. 6–15). The term "late systolic" applies to the typical murmur of mitral valve prolapse in which the murmur begins in mid to late systole and proceeds up to the aortic component of the second heart sound (see Fig. 6–6C). One or more mid to late systolic clicks often introduce the murmur (see Fig. 6–6C). The responses of the late systolic murmur and clicks to postural maneuvers (see earlier discussion) are illustrated in Figure 6–7. A *diminution* in left ventricular volume, best achieved by prompt standing after squatting[5] (see Fig. 6–34) but also achieved by the Valsalva maneuver, causes the late systolic murmur to become longer although softer. An *increase* in left ventricular volume associated with squatting or sustained handgrip causes the murmur to become shorter but louder. Pharmacologic interventions that variably alter left ventricular volume, especially amyl nitrite, produce analogous results but are less practical at the bedside.

The late systolic murmur of mitral valve prolapse is occasionally converted into an intermittent, striking late systolic whoop or honk, either spontaneously or in response to physical maneuvers. The whoop is high-frequency, musical, widely transmitted, and occasionally loud enough to be disconcertingly sensed by the patient. The musical whoop is thought to arise from mitral leaflets and chordae tendineae set into high-frequency periodic vibration. William Osler's description[19] is relevant:

> A well-nourished young girl was sent to me in May, 1888 by Dr. Buller (the first Professor of Ophthalmology at McGill University), who had noticed a remarkable whistling sound, while examining her eyes. . . . Auscultation—as she sits upright in the chair the heart sounds at the apex and base loud and clear; no murmur. When she stands, a loud systolic murmur is heard at the apex, high-pitched, somewhat musical, of maximum intensity in the fifth interspace; it varies a good deal, being loud for three or four beats, then faint for one or two succeeding ones. . . . On removal of the ear from the chest wall, the murmur can be heard at a distance of several inches. It disappeared quite suddenly and could not be detected on most careful examination. . . . The child then suggested that she heard it most frequently when in the stooping posture; on causing her to

lean forward and relax the chest, the murmur was at once heard, and with greatly increased intensity. It was distinctly audible at a distant three feet two inches by measurement, and could be heard at any point on the chest and on the top of the head.

SYSTOLIC ARTERIAL MURMURS. Detection of extracardiac systolic murmurs that originate in systemic or pulmonary arteries requires auscultation at nonprecordial sites. Systolic arterial murmurs can originate in anatomically normal arteries in the presence of normal or increased flow, or in abnormal arteries because of tortuosity or luminal narrowing. Timing with the first and second heart sounds is imprecise because these murmurs begin at variable distances from the heart. Nevertheless, the arterial murmurs dealt with here are essentially systolic and tend to have a crescendo-decrescendo configuration that reflects the rise and fall of pulsatile flow.

A normal systolic arterial murmur that is often heard in children and adolescents is called the "supraclavicular systolic murmur" (Fig. 6–26) and is believed to originate at the aortic origins of normal major brachiocephalic arteries. The configuration of these murmurs is crescendo-decrescendo, the onset abrupt, the duration brief, and at times, the intensity surprisingly loud with radiation below the clavicles. Normal supraclavicular systolic murmurs decrease or vanish in response to hypertextension of the shoulders achieved by bringing the elbows back until the shoulder girdle muscles are taut (Fig. 6–26B).

In older adults, the most common cause of a systolic arterial murmur is peripheral vascular disease that causes narrowing of carotid, subclavian, or iliofemoral arteries. Auscultation should be applied routinely over these arteries when examining older patients. A variation on this theme is a "compression artifact" in free aortic regurgitation. When a femoral artery is moderately compressed by the examiner's stethoscopic bell in a patient with severe aortic incompetence, a systolic arterial murmur is generated. Further compression can make the systolic murmur continue into diastole, a sign described in 1861 by Duroziez. The eponym is still used.

During late pregnancy, but especially in the postpartum period in lactating women, a systolic "mammary souffle"

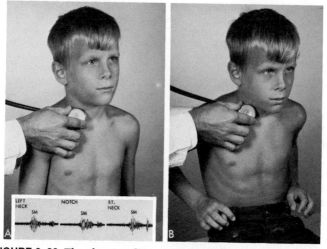

FIGURE 6–26. The phonocardiogram (*A,* inset) shows a normal supraclavicular systolic arterial murmur maximal above the clavicles (left neck, right neck) and in the suprasternal notch. Auscultation is initially carried out while the patient sits with shoulders relaxed and arms resting in the lap. *B,* When the elbows are brought well behind the back (hyperextension of the shoulders), the murmur disappears or markedly diminishes.

is sometimes heard over the breasts because of increased flow through normal arteries. The murmur begins well after the first heart sound because of the interval between left ventricular ejection and arrival of flow at the artery of origin.

Still another type of systolic arterial murmur is heard in the back over the site of coarctation of the aortic isthmus. The murmur is elicited by placing the diaphragm of the stethoscope just to the left of the vertebral column at the midthoracic level between the scapulae. Examination is best performed in infants while they are lying prone. In older children or adults, the sitting position is satisfactory provided that the thoracic muscles are relaxed.

Transient systolic arterial murmurs in the pulmonary artery and its branches are heard in occasional normal neonates because the angulation and disparity in size between the pulmonary trunk and its branches set the stage for turbulent systolic flow. These normal or innocent pulmonary arterial systolic murmurs disappear with maturation of the pulmonary bed, generally within the first few weeks or months of life. Similar if not identical pulmonary arterial systolic murmurs are heard in the axillae and back in the presence of congenital stenosis of the pulmonary artery and its branches. Rarely, a pulmonary arterial systolic murmur is caused by luminal narrowing following a pulmonary embolus.

Diastolic Murmurs (see Fig. 6–16). Murmurs in diastole are descriptively classified according to their time of *onset* as early diastolic, mid-diastolic, or late diastolic (presystolic). An *early* diastolic murmur begins with the aortic or pulmonic component of the second heart sound, depending upon its site of origin. A mid-diastolic murmur begins at a clear interval *after* the second heart sound. A late diastolic or presystolic murmur begins immediately before the first heart sound.

EARLY DIASTOLIC MURMURS (Fig. 6–16). An early diastolic murmur originating in the left side of the heart is represented by aortic regurgitation. The murmur begins with the aortic component of the second heart sound, i.e., as soon as left ventricular pressure crosses (falls below) the aortic incisura. The murmur tends to be decrescendo, reflecting the progressive decline in volume and rate of regurgitant flow during the course of diastole. Soft high-frequency early diastolic murmurs are best detected while the patient sits and leans forward in full held expiration (Fig. 6–27). In chronic free aortic regurgitation, the murmur occasionally begins with a short crescendo followed by a longer decrescendo. In moderate chronic aortic regurgitation, the aortic diastolic pressure consistently exceeds left ventricular diastolic pressure so the decrescendo is less obvious, and the murmur is well heard throughout diastole. In chronic *severe* aortic regurgitation, the decrescendo is more obvious, paralleling the dramatic decline in aortic root diastolic pressure. It is sometimes useful to determine the direction and radiation of the diastolic murmur of aortic regurgitation by comparative auscultation along the left and right sternal

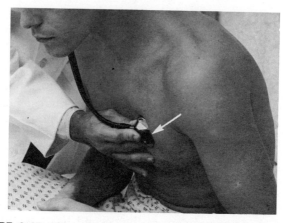

FIGURE 6–27. The soft, high-frequency early diastolic murmur of aortic regurgitation or pulmonary hypertensive pulmonary regurgitation is best elicited by applying the stethoscopic diaphragm very firmly to the mid-left sternal edge *(arrow)*. The patient leans forward with breath held in full exhalation.

borders, especially at the level of the third interspace. Selective radiation to the *right* sternal edge implies aortic root dilatation, as in the Marfan syndrome. Aortic regurgitation caused by an everted cusp often produces a distinctive musical early diastolic decrescendo murmur (Fig. 6–28). An important variation is the murmur of *acute severe* aortic regurgitation (bicuspid aortic valve infective endocarditis, dissecting aneurysm) which differs importantly from the murmur of chronic severe aortic regurgitation just described. The length (duration) of the diastolic murmur is relatively short because of early equilibration of aortic diastolic pressure with the steeply rising diastolic pressure in the poorly compliant left ventricle. The pitch of the murmur is likely to be medium and impure because the velocity of regurgitant flow is less rapid than in chronic severe aortic regurgitation. The short, medium-frequency diastolic murmur of sudden severe aortic incompetence may be disarmingly soft (grade 2/6). These auscultatory features are in contrast to the conspicuous, long, pure, high-frequency blowing diastolic murmur of *chronic* severe aortic regurgitation.

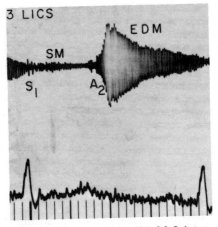

FIGURE 6–28. Phonocardiogram in the third left intercostal space (3 LICS) records the high-frequency, musical, decrescendo, early diastolic murmur (EDM) caused by eversion of an aortic cusp. S_1 = first heart sound; MS = midsystolic murmur; A_2 = aortic component of the second heart sound.

Early diastolic murmurs in the right heart are represented by the Graham Steell murmur of pulmonary hypertensive pulmonary regurgitation. The description of Steell[9] (1888) cannot be improved upon:

> I wish to plead for the admission among the recognized auscultatory signs of disease of a murmur due to pulmonary regurgitation, such regurgitation occurring independently of disease or deformity of the valves, and as a result of long-continuing excess of blood pressure in the pulmonary artery. . . . The maximum intensity of the murmur may be regarded as situated at the sternal end of the third and fourth intercostal spaces. When the second sound is reduplicated, the murmur proceeds from its latter part. That such a murmur as I have described does exist, there can, I think, be no doubt. I am prepared for the objection that the murmur under consideration is only the murmur of a slight amount of aortic regurgitation. . . . How difficult it is to distinguish between the murmurs of aortic and pulmonary regurgitation, respectively, by means of auscultation alone, will be admitted. . . . Writing in 1881, after describing the regurgitant murmur of aortic dilatation, I referred to the murmur which is the subject of this paper, as follows, 'I am inclined to believe that a murmur of similar mechanism occurs on the right side of the heart, when there is much obstruction to the pulmonary circulation, with a dilated pulmonary artery.' My subsequent expe-

rience has only served to confirm the opinion thus cautiously expressed more than 7 years ago though my faith has from time to time been shaken by a case presenting a murmur which I had at first imagined to be an example, but which, on further investigation, proved to be of aortic origin.

A Graham Steell murmur begins with the loud *pulmonic* component of the second heart sound, because the elevated pressure exerted on the incompetent pulmonic valve begins at the moment that the right ventricular pressure crosses (drops below) the pulmonary arterial incisura. The high diastolic pressure generates a high velocity of regurgitant flow and results in a high-frequency blowing murmur that may last throughout diastole. The basic configuration of the murmur is decrescendo, although occasionally the amplitude is relatively uniform throughout most if not all of diastole, and at times the murmur begins with a short crescendo. The auscultatory distinction between the early diastolic murmur of pulmonary hypertensive pulmonary regurgitation and the murmur of aortic regurgitation was underscored by Graham Steell (see above), and even today the distinction may be difficult or impossible when the pulmonic murmur is soft and the systemic arterial pulse is normal. The differentiation, if made, depends upon the clinical setting rather than upon auscultation, although squatting and sustained hand grip tend selectively to augment the murmur of aortic regurgitation (see below).

MID-DIASTOLIC MURMURS (see Fig. 6–16). Mid-diastolic murmurs begin at a clear interval after the second heart sound. The majority of mid-diastolic murmurs originate across mitral or tricuspid valves during the rapid filling phase (atrioventricular valve obstruction or abnormal patterns of atrioventricular flow) or across an incompetent pulmonic valve provided that the pulmonary arterial pressure is not elevated. Rarely, a mid-diastolic murmur is ascribed to flow through an atherosclerotic extramural coronary artery.

The mid-diastolic murmur of mitral stenosis provides a useful point of departure. The murmur may be present with sinus rhythm or atrial fibrillation and characteristically follows the mitral opening snap (Fig. 6–29A). Care

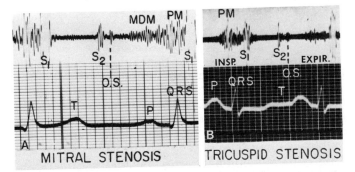

FIGURE 6–29. Phonocardiogram *(A)* recorded over the left ventricular impulse in pure rheumatic *mitral* stenosis showing the mid-diastolic murmur (MDM) followed by a presystolic murmur (PM) with crescendo up to a loud first heart sound (S_1). S_2 = second heart sound; OS = opening snap. *B,* Phonocardiogram at the fourth interspace, left sternal edge showing the presystolic murmur (PM) of rheumatic *tricuspid* stenosis. The murmur is crescendo-decrescendo, diminishing before a loud first heart sound (S_1). The first complex is during inspiration (INSP.) and finds the presystolic murmur obvious. The second complex is during expiration (EXPIR.) and finds the presystolic murmur soft. The opening snap (OS) is mitral, not tricuspid.

must be taken to place the bell of the stethoscope lightly against the skin precisely over the left ventricular impulse with the patient turned into the left lateral decubitus position (see Fig. 6–3). Because the murmur originates within the left ventricular cavity, transmission to the chest wall is maximal at the site where the left ventricle is palpated. In atrial fibrillation, the duration of the mid-diastolic murmur is a useful sign of the degree of obstruction, because a murmur that lasts up to the first heart sound even after long cycle lengths implies a persistent mitral gradient at the end of diastole. Soft mid-diastolic murmurs are reinforced when the heart rate and mitral valve flow are transiently increased by vigorous voluntary coughs.

A mid-diastolic murmur occurs with tricuspid stenosis in the presence of atrial fibrillation. The *tricuspid* mid-diastolic murmur differs from the *mitral* mid-diastolic murmur in two important respects: (1) The tricuspid murmur selectively increases in loudness during inspiration; (2) the tricuspid murmur is confined to a relatively localized area along the lower left sternal edge. The inspiratory increase in loudness occurs because inspiration is accompanied by an augmentation in right ventricular volume, by a fall in right ventricular diastolic pressure, and by an increase in the gradient and flow rate across the tricuspid valve. The murmur is localized to the lower left sternal edge because it originates within the inflow portion of the right ventricle and is transmitted to the overlying chest wall.

Mid-diastolic murmurs across *nonobstructed* atrioventricular valves occur in the presence of augmented volume and velocity of flow. Examples in the left heart are the mid-diastolic flow murmur of pure mitral regurgitation and the mid-diastolic mitral flow murmur of large left-to-right shunt ventricular septal defect. Mid-diastolic murmurs due to augmented flow across nonobstructed *tricuspid* valves are heard in severe tricuspid regurgitation or in the presence of a large left-to-right shunt ostium secundum atrial septal defect. These mid-diastolic flow murmurs, whether mitral or tricuspid, are typically short and medium-pitched, tend to occur with appreciable atrioventricular valve incompetence or large shunts, and are often preceded by third heart sounds, especially in the presence of mitral or tricuspid regurgitation.

In complete heart block, short, mid-diastolic atrioventricular flow murmurs sometimes occur when atrial contraction coincides with the phase of rapid diastolic filling. These murmurs are believed to result from antegrade flow across atrioventricular valves that are closing rapidly during filling of the recipient ventricle. A similar mechanism has been assigned to the Austin Flint murmur, as Flint originally described[20] (see below).

A mid-diastolic murmur is a feature of pulmonary valve regurgitation provided that the pulmonary arterial pressure is normal or low (Fig. 6–30A). The cause of the pulmonary regurgitation can be present at birth (congenital) or acquired (pulmonic valve infective endocarditis in intravenous drug abusers). The most common cause of low pressure pulmonary valve regurgitation, however, is surgical repair of obstructive lesions of the right ventric-

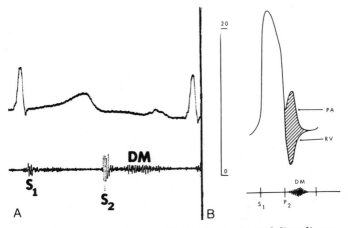

FIGURE 6–30. Phonocardiogram *(A)* illustrating the mid-diastolic murmur (MDM) of low-pressure pulmonary valve regurgitation in a heroin addict with pulmonary valve infective endocarditis. The murmur begins well after the second sound (S₂), is medium-frequency, mid-diastolic, and ends well before the subsequent first heart sound (S₁). *B,* Pressure pulses and phonocardiogram illustrate the physiologic mechanism of the mid-diastolic murmur (MDM) of low-pressure pulmonary regurgitation. Because the pressure exerted against the incompetent pulmonic valve is low, the murmur does not begin until well after the right ventricular (RV) and pulmonary arterial (PA) pressure pulses diverge. The murmur is maximal when the diastolic gradient (cross-hatched area) is greatest. (Note the early diastolic dip in the RV pulse.) Equilibration of the pulmonary arterial and right ventricular pressures in later diastole abolishes the regurgitant gradient, so the murmur disappears.

ular outflow tract. The accompanying diastolic murmur typically begins at a perceptible interval after the pulmonic component of the second heart sound and is crescendo-decrescendo ending well before the subsequent second heart sound.

The physiologic mechanism responsible for the timing of the murmur of low-pressure pulmonary regurgitation is shown in Figure 6–30B. The diastolic pressure exerted upon the incompetent pulmonic valve is negligible at the time of the pulmonic component of the second heart sound, so regurgitant flow is minimal at that instant. Regurgitation accelerates as the right ventricular pressure dips below the diastolic pressure in the pulmonary trunk; at that point the murmur reaches its maximum (Fig. 6–30B). Late diastolic equilibration of pulmonary arterial and right ventricular pressures eliminates regurgitant flow and abolishes the murmur prior to the next first heart sound. When the pulmonic component of the second sound is late, soft, or absent, an even more conspicuous gap exists between the aortic component and the onset of the pulmonic diastolic murmur.

LATE DIASTOLIC OR PRESYSTOLIC MURMURS. A late diastolic murmur occurs immediately before the first heart sound, that is, in *presystole*. The late diastolic timing coincides with the period of ventricular filling that follows atrial systole and implies coordinated atrial contraction, generally sinus rhythm. Late diastolic or presystolic murmurs can originate at the mitral or tricuspid orifice, usually because of obstruction, but occasionally because of abnormal patterns of presystolic atrioventricular flow.

The most celebrated presystolic murmur accompanies rheumatic mitral stenosis in sinus rhythm as atrioventricular flow is augmented by an increase in the force of left atrial systole (Fig. 6–29A). Moderate "presystolic" accentuation of a mid-diastolic murmur is occasionally heard in mitral stenosis with atrial fibrillation, especially during short cycle lengths, but the timing is actually early systolic, and the mechanism differs from the true presystolic murmur shown in Figure 6–29A. The technique for eliciting or reinforcing the presystolic murmur of mitral stenosis is the same as that described above for the mitral mid-diastolic murmur.

In *tricuspid* stenosis with sinus rhythm, a late diastolic or presystolic murmur characteristically occurs in the absence of a perceptible mid-diastolic murmur (Fig. 6–29B). This is so because the timing of tricuspid diastolic murmurs coincides with the maximal acceleration of flow and gradient, which are usually negligible until the powerful right atrium contracts. The presystolic murmur of tricuspid stenosis is crescendo-decrescendo in shape and rather discrete, fading in decrescendo toward the first heart sound (Fig. 6–29B), in contrast to the presystolic murmur of mitral stenosis which tends to rise in crescendo to the first heart sound (Fig. 6–29A). However, the most valuable auscultatory sign of tricuspid stenosis in sinus rhythm is the effect of respiration on the presystolic murmur. Inspiration increases right atrial volume, provoking an increase in right atrial contractile force in the face of a fall in right ventricular end-diastolic pressure. The result is a larger gradient, an increased velocity of tricuspid flow, and an increase in the intensity of the tricuspid stenotic presystolic murmur, as shown in Figure 6–29B.

Presystolic and mid-diastolic murmurs occasionally occur in patients with a myxoma of the left or right atrium. These murmurs may resemble the murmurs of mitral or tricuspid stenosis, and the "tumor plop" (see above) may be mistaken for an opening snap.

In complete heart block, short, crescendo-decrescendo presystolic murmurs are occasionally heard when atrial contraction fortuitously falls in late diastole. However, the diastolic murmur in complete heart block is usually mid-diastolic (see above) when atrial contraction coincides with and reinforces the rapid filling phase.

The Austin Flint presystolic murmur was described in 1862,[20] and the mechanism proposed by Flint was astonishingly perceptive:

> Is this murmur ever produced without any mitral lesions? One would a priori suppose the answer of this question to be in the negative. Clinical observation, however, shows that the question is to be answered in the affirmative. . . . In May, 1860, I examined a patient, age 56. . . . At the apex was a pre-systolic blubbering murmur. . . .

At necropsy, three days later,

> The aorta was atheromatous and dilated so as to render the valvular segments evidently insufficient. The mitral valve presented nothing abnormal. . . .

Flint examined a second case the following year and concluded:

> In both cases the mitral direct murmur was loud and had that character of sound which I supposed to be due to vibration of the mitral curtains. In both cases it will be observed, an aortic regurgitant murmur existed, and aortic insufficiency was found to exist at

postmortem. . . . A mitral direct murmur, then, may exist without mitral contraction and without any mitral lesions, provided there be aortic lesions involving considerable aortic regurgitation.

Flint then proposed the following mechanism:

Now in cases of considerable aortic insufficiency, the left ventricle is rapidly filled with blood flowing back from the aorta as well as from the auricle, before the auricular contraction takes place. The distention of the ventricle is such that the mitral curtains are brought into coaptation, and when the auricular contraction takes place the mitral direct current passing between the curtains throws them into vibration and gives rise to the characteristic blubbering murmur.

Austin Flint was one of the most distinguished physicians of nineteenth century American medicine. He has been called "America's Laënnec."[21]

Presystolic murmurs tend to be relatively low to medium in frequency, so auscultation should be conducted with just enough pressure of the bell of the stethoscope to achieve a skin seal. Presystolic murmurs originating across the mitral valve are best elicited over the left ventricular impulse with the patient in a partial left lateral decubitus position. Presystolic murmurs across the tricuspid valve are best elicited with the patient supine while the examiner applies the stethoscope to the lower left sternal edge, moving the bell in small increments in search of the localized murmur. A presystolic tricuspid murmur, especially of tricuspid stenosis, may be heard *only* during inspiration (see Fig. 6–29*B*), so the patient should be instructed to breathe in and then breathe out rhythmically and with a moderate increase in depth.

Continuous Murmurs (see Fig. 6–17). The term "continuous" is applied to murmurs that begin in systole and continue without interruption through the timing of the second heart sound into all or part of diastole. Accordingly, the presence of murmurs that fill both phases of the cardiac cycle (holosystolic followed by holodiastolic, see Fig. 6–17) is not a requirement. Conversely, a murmur that fades completely before the subsequent first heart sound is continuous provided that the murmur that begins in systole proceeds without interruption through the timing of the second heart sound (see Fig. 6–17).

Continuous murmurs generally occur when there is

flow from a zone of higher resistance into a zone of lower resistance without phasic interruption between systole and diastole. Such murmurs are due chiefly to (1) aortopulmonary connections, (2) arteriovenous connections, (3) disturbances of flow patterns in arteries, and (4) disturbances of flow patterns in veins (see Fig. 6–17).

The best-known continuous murmur is associated with patent ductus arteriosus (Figs. 6–17 and 6–31). This aortopulmonary continuous murmur characteristically peaks just before and after the second heart sound and is often soft or even absent in late diastole before the subsequent first heart sound. In 1847, the *London Medical Gazette* published the description of "a murmur accompanying the first heart sound . . . prolonged into the second so that there is no cessation of the murmur before the second sound has already commenced."[22] The author not only correctly assigned the cause of the murmur to patent ductus arteriosus but also established the true meaning of "continuous" as "no cessation of the murmur before the second sound has already commenced." In

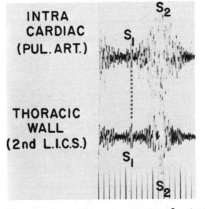

FIGURE 6–31. The classic continuous murmur of patent ductus arteriosus recorded from within the main pulmonary artery (PUL. ART.) and simultaneously at the second left intercostal space on the thoracic wall (2 LICS). The murmur "begins softly and increases in intensity so as to reach its acme just about, or immediately after the incidence of the second sound, and from that point gradually wanes until its termination," as originally described by Gibson in 1900.

1900, George A. Gibson[23] provided us with an accurate and meticulous description of the murmur of patent ductus arteriosus that is still called the "Gibson murmur." He wrote: "It persists through the second sound and dies away gradually during the long pause. The murmur is rough and thrilling. It begins softly and increases in intensity so as to reach its acme just about, or immediately after, the incidence of the second sound, and from that point gradually wanes until its termination." The description cannot be improved upon (Fig. 6–31).

Arteriovenous continuous murmurs can be congenital or acquired and are represented in part by arteriovenous fistulas, coronary arterial fistulas, anomalous origin of the left coronary artery from the pulmonary trunk, and sinus of Valsalva to right heart communications. The configuration, location, and intensity of arteriovenous continuous murmurs vary considerably among these different categories. The continuous murmur due to a systemic arteriovenous fistula was described by Josef Skoda. The English translation reads: "When a moderately sized artery communicates with a vein, a very loud continuous murmur usually develops at the point of communication, the strength of which increases on each pulsation of the artery and is audible over a greater or lesser part of the surrounding area."[24] *Acquired* systemic arteriovenous fistulas are commonly represented by surgically produced forearm arteriovenous connections used for chronic renal dialysis. The continuous murmur of a *congenital* coronary arterial fistula that enters the right ventricle can be either softer or louder in systole, depending upon the degree of compression exerted upon the fistulous coronary artery by right ventricular contraction. The murmur accompanying ruptured sinus of Valsalva aneurysm into the right heart is continuous but does not peak before and after the second heart sound, tending instead to be louder in either systole or diastole, sometimes creating a to-and-fro impression.

Arterial continuous murmurs originate in either *constricted* or *nonconstricted* arteries. Continuous disturbances of flow in constricted systemic or pulmonary arteries occur when a significant and continuous difference in pressure exists between the two sides of the narrowed segment. Arterial continuous murmurs arising in constricted arteries are characteristically louder in systole (see Fig. 6–17). Common examples are represented by atherosclerotic carotid or femoral arterial obstruction.

Disturbances of flow patterns in *normal, nonconstricted* arteries sometimes produce continuous murmurs. The "mammary souffle" (see above) is an innocent murmur heard during late pregnancy and the puerperium and is sometimes continuous. These continuous arterial murmurs are typically louder in systole (see Fig. 6–17) and are maximal over either lactating breast. There is a tendency, however, for the murmur to be somewhat louder in the second or third right or left intercostal space. A distinct gap separates the first heart sound from the onset of the mammary souffle because of the interval that must elapse before blood ejected from the left ventricle arrives at the artery of origin. The mammary souffle is best heard with the patient supine. The souffle sometimes vanishes altogether in the upright position. Light pressure with the stethoscope tends to augment the murmur and bring out its continuous features, whereas firm pressure with the stethoscope or by digital compression peripheral to the site of auscultation often abolishes the murmur.

Continuous murmurs in nonconstricted arteries can originate in the large systemic to pulmonary arterial collaterals in certain types of cyanotic congenital heart disease, especially Fallot's tetralogy with pulmonary atresia. These continuous murmurs must be diligently sought, because they are randomly located throughout the thorax.

Continuous venous murmurs are epitomized by the innocent venous hum (Fig. 6–32). The hum is by far the most common type of normal continuous murmur, almost universal in healthy children, and frequently present in healthy young adults, especially during pregnancy. Potain described the venous hum in 1867:

> The thrill, which is felt by placing the finger lightly above the clavicle over the course of the vessel of the neck, is sometimes continuous and frequently intermittent. It is this last case which interests us above all here. . . . A light pressure exerted above the point of exploration can make it appear or reinforce it, while a

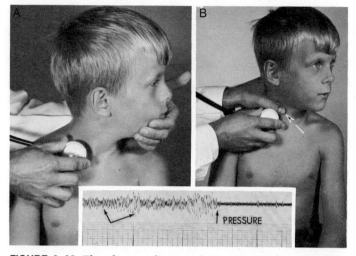

FIGURE 6–32. The phonocardiogram shows the continuous murmur of a normal venous hum. The *diastolic* component of the murmur is louder *(paired arrows)*. Digital pressure over the right internal jugular vein *(vertical arrow)* obliterates the murmur. The accompanying two photographs show maneuvers used to elicit or abolish the venous hum. *A,* The bell of the stethoscope is applied to the medial aspect of the right supraclavicular fossa. The examiner's left hand grasps the patient's chin from behind and pulls it tautly to the left and upward, stretching the neck. *B,* Digital compression of the right internal jugular vein *(arrow)* obliterates the hum. The patient's head has returned to a more neutral position.

> stronger pressure extinguishes it completely, proofs positive . . .
> that we are concerned with a venous phenomenon and that this
> thrill does not arise at all from an artery.[25]

The venous hum is elicited with the patient in the sitting position (Fig. 6–32). The stethoscopic bell is applied to the medial aspect of the right supraclavicular fossa, while the examiner's left hand grasps the patient's chin from behind and pulls it tautly to the left and upward (Fig. 6–32A). The hum generally disappears by removing the "stretch" on the neck as the head is returned to a relatively neutral position (Fig. 6–32B). Occasionally, the hum appears or increases when the chin is simply tilted upward, and at other times it is prominent without neck maneuvers and irrespective of position. Venous hums in young children may come and go when the child turns its head to the left or looks upward. The simplest and most effective procedure for abolishing the hum is application of pressure to the deep jugular vein with the thumb of the examiner's free hand as Potain described and as shown in Figure 6–32B. Compression typically causes instantaneous disappearance of the hum (see phonocardiographic insert, Fig. 6–32B), which suddenly but transiently intensifies as pressure is released. The term "hum" does not necessarily describe the quality of these cervical venous continuous murmurs, which may be rough, noisy, or accompanied by a high-pitched whine. The venous hum is truly continuous and characteristically louder in diastole (Fig. 6–32), as is the case with venous continuous murmurs in general (see Fig. 6–17). Radiation of a loud venous hum below the clavicles sets the stage for a mistaken diagnosis of an intrathoracic continuous murmur. Obliteration by digital pressure in the neck abolishes the transmitted hum and avoids error.

PERICARDIAL RUBS

Pericardial rubs are heard in systole (generally midsystole), mid-diastole, and late diastole (presystole). In sinus rhythm, the classic rub is triple-phased, i.e., midsystolic, mid-diastolic, and presystolic. Diagnosis is simplest when all three phases are present and when the typical superficial, scratchy, leathery quality is evident. Rubs are most readily detected at the mid to lower left sternal edge when the stethoscopic diaphragm is firmly applied during full held expiration. If doubt persists, the precordium can then be examined with the patient resting on elbows and knees, a position designed to promote apposition of visceral and parietal pericardium (Fig. 6–33). The systolic phase of a rub is the most consistent, followed by the presystolic phase. In atrial fibrillation, the presystolic component necessarily disappears. The diagnosis of a pericardial rub is least secure, and often impossible, when only one phase remains, which is, as a rule, midsystolic

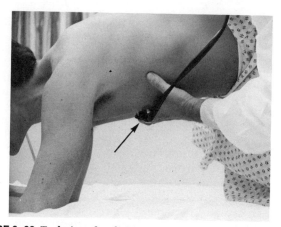

FIGURE 6–33. Technique for eliciting a pericardial rub. The diaphragm of the stethoscope is firmly applied to the precordium *(arrow)* while the patient rests on elbows and knees.

but occasionally presystolic. The most common clinical setting in which pericardial rubs occur is immediately following open heart surgery. However, auscultation in the immediate postoperative period may detect instead a crunching noise synchronous with the heartbeat heard over the cardiac apex in the left lateral decubitus position. This is Hamman's sign caused by air in the mediastinum.

PHYSICAL MANEUVERS

A number of the physical maneuvers employed during auscultation have already been discussed. The following remarks emphasize the importance of these maneuvers by bringing most if not all of them briefly into focus (Tables 6–5 and 6–6). I shall not deal with pharmacologic interventions, except for amyl nitrite inhalation, because they are of less practical importance at the bedside.

Changes in position that are useful during auscultation are listed in Table 6–5. A partial left lateral decubitus position (see Fig. 6–3) assists in identifying the left ventricular impulse, which is an important auscultatory

TABLE 6–5. Changes in Position During Auscultation

Left lateral decubitus
Sitting, leaning forward
Sitting with legs dangling
Standing to squatting and vice versa
Hyperextension of the shoulders
"Stretching" of the neck
Passive elevation of the legs
Elevation of precordium on elbows and knees

site. During the act of turning, the heart rate sometimes transiently increases, improving audibility of mid-diastolic and presystolic murmurs of mitral stenosis. The left lateral decubitus position occasionally induces premature ventricular beats that may assist in distinguishing an aortic midsystolic murmur heard at the apex from the apical murmur of mitral regurgitation.

Sitting and leaning forward in full held expiration (see Fig. 6–27) helps in detecting the soft, high-frequency early diastolic murmur of aortic regurgitation or the Graham Steell murmur. Sitting with legs dangling aids in establishing normal splitting of the second heart sound when the split fails to fuse during expiration in the supine position.

The sequence of standing and squatting followed by prompt standing (Figs. 6–7 and 6–34) is best done with the patient's examining gown removed or securely fastened so the garment doesn't fall from the shoulders and interfere with the auscultatory examination. During the squatting/standing maneuver, balance is important, especially in older adults, who should squat within arm's reach of the edge of the bed or examining table for support (Fig. 6–34). Standing, squatting, and prompt standing are

TABLE 6–6. Other Physical Maneuvers During Auscultation

Respiration
  Inspiration, expiration
  Full, held expiration
Valsalva and Müller maneuvers
Isometric (handgrip) and isotonic (dynamic) exercise
Vigorous coughing

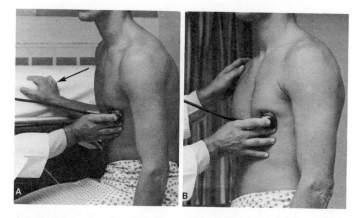

FIGURE 6–34. Auscultation during squatting *(A)* and prompt standing *(B)*. The maneuvers are best done in that sequence. The patient should use the right hand for support by holding the edge of the bed or examining table *(arrow)*.

useful maneuvers in assessing the murmurs of aortic and mitral regurgitation, mitral valve prolapse, and hypertrophic obstructive cardiomyopathy.

Hyperextension of the shoulders is an important positional maneuver in assessing supraclavicular systolic murmurs (Fig. 6–26). For initiating or reinforcing a venous hum, the patient's neck should be stretched upward and to the left as the stethoscope is applied to the medial aspect of the right supraclavicular fossa (see Fig. 6–32).

Passive elevation of both legs with the patient supine and horizontal transiently increases venous return and augments third heart sounds. The patient must be instructed not to assist in the leg raising. This precaution avoids involuntary straining and a partial Valsalva maneuver.

From the prone position, the precordium can be elevated above the bed or examining table by having the patient rise on the elbows and knees (see Fig. 6–33). This maneuver assists in detecting pericardial friction rubs.

Physical maneuvers other than positional changes (Table 6–6) also aid in auscultation. *Respiration* is routinely employed in the form of normal inspiration and expiration. Normal or exaggerated respiratory excursions are useful for analysis of splitting of the second heart sound, right-sided third and fourth heart sounds, tricuspid systolic and diastolic murmurs, and pulmonic ejection sounds. The examiner can instruct the patient on the desired pattern of respiration by illustrating the required depth and rate of breathing. Full held expiration is employed when searching for the soft, early diastolic murmur of aortic regurgitation or pulmonary hypertensive pulmonary regurgitation while the patient sits and leans forward (see Fig. 6–27). A subtle pericardial friction rub may be heard during held exhalation while the patient is supine. The innocent pulmonic midsystolic murmur associated with decreased anteroposterior chest dimensions (loss of thoracic kyphosis) may dramatically amplify when the diaphragm of the stethoscope is pressed firmly in the second left intercostal space during full held expiration.

The Valsalva maneuver can be readily performed at the bedside and consists of a deep inspiration followed by forced expiration against a closed glottis for 10 to 12 seconds. The Valsalva maneuver was described in 1704 as a method for expelling pus from the middle ear by straining (expiration) with the mouth and nose closed. The patient should be instructed on how to perform the maneuver. Simulation by the examiner is a simple means of doing so. The examiner then places the flat of the hand upon the abdomen to provide the patient with a force against which to strain and to permit assessment of the degree and duration of the straining effort. The normal Valsalva response consists of four phases. *Phase 1* is associated with a transient rise in systemic blood pressure as straining begins. This phase cannot, as a rule, be identified at the bedside. *Phase 2* is accompanied by a perceptible decrease in blood pressure and pulse pressure (small pulse) and a readily detectable reflex tachycardia. *Phase 3* begins with cessation of straining and is associated with an abrupt, transient decrease in blood pressure. This phase is generally not perceived at the bedside and is followed promptly by *Phase 4*, which is characterized by an overshoot of systemic arterial pressure and relatively obvious reflex bradycardia.

The Müller maneuver is the converse of the Valsalva maneuver but is less frequently employed because it is less useful at the bedside. The maneuver is performed for about 10 seconds as the patient forcibly inspires while the nares are held closed and the mouth is firmly sealed. By exaggerating the inspiratory effort, the Müller maneuver occasionally augments the murmur of tricuspid regurgitation or stenosis, but the usefulness of the maneuver is limited.

Isometric exercise (sustained handgrip) is a useful, simple, safe maneuver that can be performed in a few minutes at the bedside. The normal response to sustained handgrip is an increase in systolic blood pressure, an increase in left ventricular systolic pressure and end-diastolic pressure, and an increase in heart rate and cardiac index with prompt return to control values upon cessation of the maneuver. To achieve the desired effect of isometric exercise, it is usually sufficient to instruct the patient merely to squeeze both empty fists simultaneously, but if the fingernails are long, a small, firm rubber ball or analogous object can be compressed. Care should be taken to have the patient clench the fists without tensing the proximal muscle groups, especially the shoulder girdle. Sustained handgrip is maintained until the examiner tells the patient to desist. The duration of handgrip depends in part upon when and whether a positive auscultatory response is elicited. Auscultation should therefore precede, accompany, and follow the maneuver, which can cease if the sought-for auscultatory response is elicited. Twenty seconds of maximum isometric exercise are more than sufficient. The physiologic response to sustained handgrip reinforces left ventricular fourth heart sounds; the murmurs of mitral and aortic regurgitation get louder. The click(s) of mitral valve prolapse occur later in systole, and the late systolic murmur shortens but increases in intensity. The systolic murmur of hypertrophic obstructive cardiomyopathy decreases in response to the isometric exercise of sustained handgrip.

Amyl nitrite inhalation occasionally has a place during

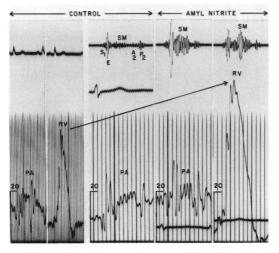

FIGURE 6–35. Tracings from a teenager with mild pulmonic valve stenosis (control gradient 25 mm Hg). Following amyl nitrite inhalation, the right ventricular (RV) pressure rose *(arrow)*, the gradient increased, and an initially short, soft systolic murmur (SM) became louder and longer. E = pulmonic ejection sound; PA = pulmonary arterial pulse.

auscultation. The drug results in prompt falls in systemic vascular resistance and blood pressure and an increase in heart rate, cardiac output, and ejection velocity. The room in which the drug is administered should be well ventilated. Amyl nitrite is inhaled from a broken vial held close to the patient's nose, preferably under a small cloth or handkerchief. The patient is instructed to breathe naturally while the examiner carefully monitors the arterial pulse rate for the first evidence of reflex tachycardia. Inhalation is discontinued as soon as the pulse begins to accelerate, a response which indicates that systemic resistance has fallen. The pulse rate is a simpler and better monitor than the cuff blood pressure, and the response to inhalation during continuous natural breathing is easier to monitor than the response to several rapid deep breaths.

The auscultatory effects of amyl nitrite inhalation are in accord with the hemodynamic effects just described.

An increase in cardiac output and ejection velocity is accompanied by an increase in loudness of the systolic murmur of aortic stenosis or of isolated pulmonic stenosis (Fig. 6–35). A decrease in systemic vascular resistance is accompanied by a decrease in the systolic murmur of mitral regurgitation and in the diastolic murmur of aortic regurgitation. The mid to late systolic clicks and late systolic murmur of mitral valve prolapse occur earlier (reduction in left ventricular volume), but the murmur becomes softer (decreased resistance to left ventricular discharge). In hypertrophic obstructive cardiomyopathy, the systolic murmur intensifies because amyl nitrite causes a decrease in left ventricular volume and an increase in ejection velocity.

REFERENCES

1. Stokes, W.: An Introduction to the Use of the Stethoscope. Edinburgh, Maclachlan and Stewart, 1825.
2. Craige, E.: Should auscultation be rehabilitated? N. Engl. J. Med. 318:1611, 1988.
3. Latham, P. M.: Lectures on Subjects Connected with Clinical Medicine Comprising Diseases of the Heart. Philadelphia, Barrington and Hoswell, 1847.
4. Laënnec, R. T. H.: A Treatise on the Diseases of the Chest (translated by John Forbes). Philadelphia, James Webster, 1823.
5. Lembo, N. J., Dell'Italia, L. J., Crawford, M. H., and O'Rourke, R. A.: Bedside diagnosis of systolic murmurs. N. Engl. J. Med. 318:1572, 1988.
6. Potain, P. C.: Clinique médicale de la Charité. Paris, Masson, 1894. *In* McKusick, V. A.: Cardiovascular Sound in Health and Disease. Baltimore, The Williams & Wilkins Company, 1958.
7. Leatham, A.: The second heart sound. Key to auscultation of the heart. Acta Cardiol. 19:395, 1964.
8. Potain, P. C.: Note sur les dédoublements normaux des bruits du coeur. Bull. Mem. Soc. Med. Hop. Paris 3:138, 1866.
9. Steell, G.: The murmur of high-pressure in the pulmonary artery. Med. Chron. Manchester 9:182, 1888–1899.
10. Connolly, D. C., and Mann, R. J.: Dominic J. Corrigan (1802–1880) and his description of the pericardial knock. Mayo Clin. Proc. 55:771, 1980.
11. Potain, P. C.: Concerning the cardiac rhythm called gallop rhythm. Bull. Mem. Soc. Med. Hop. Paris 12:137, 1876. *In* Major, R. H.: Classic Descriptions of Disease. 3rd ed. Springfield, Illinois, Charles C Thomas, Publisher, 1948.

12. Ozawa, M. D., Smith, D., and Craige, E.: Origin of the third heart sound. Circulation 678:399, 1983.
13. Freeman, A. R., and Levine, S. A.: The clinical significance of the systolic murmur. A study of 1000 consecutive "non-cardiac" cases. Ann. Intern. Med. 6:1371, 1933.
14. Leatham, A.: Auscultation of the heart. Lancet 2:703, 1958.
15. Gallavardin, L., and Pauper-Ravault. Le souffle du rétrécissement aortique peut changer de timbre et devenir musical dans sa propagation apexienne. Lyon Med., 1925, p. 523.
16. Stokes, W.: Diseases of the Heart and Aorta. Philadelphia, Lindsay and Blakiston, 1855.
17. Still, G. F.: Common Disorders and Diseases of Childhood. London, Henry Frowde, 1909.
18. Rivero-Carvallo, J. M.: Signo para el diagnostico de las insuficiencias tricuspideas. Arch. Inst. Cardiol. Mex. 16:531, 1946.
19. Osler, W.: On a remarkable heart murmur, heard at a distance from the chest wall. Med. Times Gaz. Lond. 2:432, 1880.
20. Flint, A.: On cardiac murmurs. Am. J. Med. Sci. 44:23, 1862.
21. Berman, P.: Austin Flint—America's Laënnec revisited. Arch. Intern. Med. 148:2053, 1988.
22. Williams, X.: Comment in discussion of case of patent ductus arteriosus with aortic valve disease, coarctation of aorta and infective endocarditis reported by Babington. Lond. Med. Gaz. 4:822, 1847.
23. Gibson, G. A.: Persistence of the arterial duct and its diagnosis. Edinb. Med. J. 8:1, 1900.
24. Skoda, J.: Abhandlung uber Perkussion und Auskultation. Vienna, L. W. Seidl und John. Sechste Auflage, 1864.
25. Potain, P. C.: Des mouvements et de bruits qui se passent dans les veines jugulaires. Bull. Mem. Soc. Med. Hop. Paris 4:3, 1867.

THE CHEST

The pulmonary circulation was discovered by Michael Servetus (1509–1553), a Portuguese scholar who was burned at the stake by Calvin. Gian Alfonso Borelli (1608–1679), applying the laws of mechanics, called attention to the importance of intercostal muscles and the diaphragm in respiration. The relationship between the pulmonary circulation and respiration makes it axiomatic that the physical examination of the heart and circulation include an assessment of the chest—its physical appearance and respiratory movements, together with palpation, percussion, and auscultation. Physical appearance of the thorax was dealt with in Chapter 2. This chapter focuses on respiratory movements, palpation, percussion, and auscultation of the chest.

Observation of the *pattern of respiratory movements* should be done without making the patient conscious of the examiner's intent; i.e., the patient should not be instructed to "breathe normally." The observed pattern depends in part upon the position that the patient assumes for the greatest ease of breathing. Orthopnea (*orthos* = straight; *pnoia* = breath) implies that the most comfortable position is straight or semiupright. Trepopnea (*trepein* = to turn; *pnoia* = breath) refers to a condition in which breathing is easiest with the patient turned into a recumbent position lying on one side.

Once the patient has selected the most comfortable position, the frequency and depth of respiration should be noted. Respiratory frequency, all else being equal, is in part age related. The relatively rapid and somewhat

249

irregular breathing of the normal newborn contrasts with the slower rhythmic breathing of the adult. Respiratory excursions can be abnormally slow (bradypnea) or abnormally rapid (tachypnea) or may transiently cease altogether (apnea). The depth of each respiratory excursion can be excessive (hyperpnea) or shallow, and hyperpnea can be persistent (the Kussmaul breathing of metabolic acidosis) or episodic (intermittent, deep sighing hyperventilatory excursions). Inspiration and expiration may be effortless or may be labored and prolonged. A few examples suffice.

Tachypnea typically announces heart failure in infants and is followed by labored respiration manifested chiefly by an inspiratory effort that uses accessory muscles and produces subcostal and suprasternal retraction. In adults, the tachypnea of acute pulmonary edema is accompanied by noisy inspiratory and expiratory gurgling, a cough that is productive of pink, frothy sputum, flaring alae nasi, and labored use of accessory muscles of respiration. Tachypnea is a common and sometimes insidious sign of submassive pulmonary embolism.

Periodic breathing takes different forms, among the most common of which is the deep, sighing inspiratory effort of psychophysiologic hyperventilatory dyspnea in otherwise normal but anxious patients. Single deep inspiratory sighs are accompanied by the feeling of an unfulfilled, less than satisfying breath. A celebrated type of periodic breathing was described by William Stokes[1] and later came to be known as Cheyne-Stokes respiration. Stokes's description cannot be improved upon.

> The decline in the length and force of the respirations is as regular and remarkable as their progressive increase. The inspirations become each one less deep than the preceding, until they are all but imperceptible, and then the state of apparent apnoea occurs. This is at last broken by the faintest possible inspiration; the next effort is a little stronger, until, so to speak, the paroxysm is at its height, again to subside by a descending scale.

A tracing of Cheyne-Stokes respiration recorded by James Mackenzie on his polygraph is shown in Figure 7–1.

One of the most colorful accounts of periodic breathing is C. Sidney Burwell's report of the pickwickian syn-

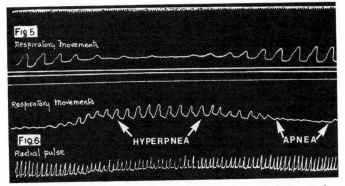

FIGURE 7–1. "Respiratory movements from a case of Cheyne-Stokes respiration" recorded by James Mackenzie.[2] (Arrows and labels are mine.)

drome. Periods of apnea during involuntary sleep (Fig. 7–2) alternate with periods of tachypnea that suddenly awaken the patient. Charles Dickens observed diseases with the eye of an expert clinician; Burwell's story does credit to a novelist. In describing a 51-year-old business executive who was hospitalized because of obesity, fatigue, and somnolence, Burwell wrote: "The patient was accustomed to playing poker once a week, and on the crucial occasion he was dealt a hand of three aces and two kings. According to Hoyle, this hand is called a 'full house.' *Because he had dropped off to sleep, he failed to take advantage of this opportunity.* A few days later, he entered the Peter Bent Brigham Hospital."[3]

Pulmonary emphysema with chronic obstructive lung disease is accompanied by distinctive patterns of thoracic movement. The respiratory muscles, especially the diaphragm, are among the only skeletal muscles upon which life literally depends. William Stokes wrote in 1825: "When respiration is produced by the intercostal, and other respiratory muscles, it is called *thoracic*; when by the action of the diaphragm alone, *abdominal*." During quiet normal breathing in the supine position, most of the respiratory movements are abdominal, while in the upright position, there is considerably more rib motion. The relative contributions of thoracic and abdominal

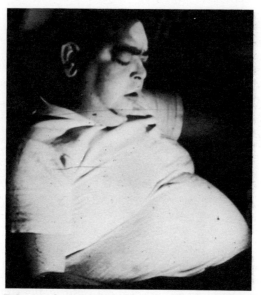

FIGURE 7–2. An obese 32-year-old man with the pickwickian syndrome photographed by the author as the patient fell asleep while his history was being taken.

muscles can be established by simple bedside observation. The assessment of *inspiratory* muscle function aids in the physical diagnosis of pulmonary emphysema. The hyperinflated lungs (Fig. 7–3) materially compromise if not eliminate the diaphragmatic contribution to breathing because the crural portions of the hemidiaphragms are flattened, thus shortening their inspiratory muscle fiber length. Accordingly, rib-cage muscles are recruited to assist the diaphragm in its task.[4] These accessory thoracic respiratory muscles literally lift the sternum with each breath, a movement that coincides with brisk inward excursion of the abdomen. This distinctive "see-saw" pattern of thoracic and abdominal motion is best observed from the foot of the bed. *Expiration* in the emphysematous patient is forced and prolonged, often through pursed lips, and is accompanied by tensing of abdominal muscles and distention of neck veins that collapse briskly during

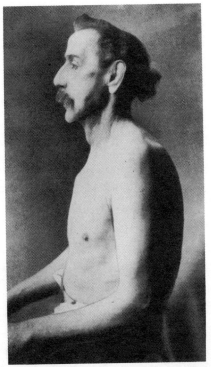

FIGURE 7–3. "Barrel chest due to chronic bronchitis and emphysema." (From Cabot, R. C.: Physical Diagnosis. New York, William Wood and Co, 1915. Courtesy of Dr. Sherman M. Mellinkoff, UCLA Medical Center.)

the subsequent labored inspiration. Patients often sit and lean forward with arms extended for support.

Palpation of the thorax, apart from and in addition to movements imparted by the heart and great arteries (see Chapter 5), falls into two categories—tactile fremitus and pressure applied to elicit local musculoskeletal tenderness. Tactile fremitus refers to vibrations perceptible on palpation and elicited by placing the ulnar side of the hand or the fingertips against the chest wall and instructing the patient to say "ninety-nine" in a relatively loud deep voice. Tactile fremitus is increased by lung consolidation and decreased by overexpansion of the lung as in pulmonary emphysema (Fig. 7–3).

Locally applied pressure serves to elicit musculoskeletal tenderness that sometimes clarifies noncardiac chest pain. With the patient supine, pressure is selectively applied with the fingertips over each chondrosternal junction, comparing the left to the right. Pain elicited over a costal cartilage, generally to the left of the sternum, has been called "Tietze's syndrome." In addition, localized left submammary pain is occasionally accompanied by a circumscribed area of submammary tenderness. In evaluating the chest for tenderness, it is sometimes recommended that the patient's back be struck gently with the fist, a procedure that I seldom use.

Let us now turn to *percussion* of the human thorax, a technique discovered by Leopold Auenbrugger[5] (Fig. 7–4),

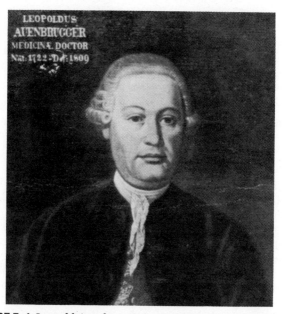

FIGURE 7–4. Leopold Auenbrugger (1722–1809). (Courtesy of Kathleen Donohue, Director, Special Collections Division, Biomedical Library, UCLA Medical Center.)

and heralded as the beginning of modern clinical diagnosis. "The method of *Percussion* is founded on the property possessed by the human thorax, in common with most hollow bodies, of giving out certain sounds when struck in a particular manner."[5] Let Auenbrugger speak for himself through the Forbes translation of "Inventum Novum ex Percussione Thoracis Humani."[5]

> I here present the reader with a new sign which I have discovered for detecting diseases of the chest. This consists in percussion of the human thorax, whereby, according to the character of the particular sounds thence elicited, an opinion is formed of the internal state of that cavity.
>
> The sound thus elicited from the healthy chest, resembles the stifled sound of a drum covered with a thick woolen cloth or other envelop (envelope) . . . . To be able justly to appreciate the value of the various sounds elicted from the chest in cases of disease, it is necessary to have learned by experience on many subjects, the modification of sound . . . produced by the habit of the body . . . inasmuch as these various circumstances modify the sound very considerably . . . . A clear and equal sound solicited from both sides of the chest indicates that the air cells of the lungs are free, and uncompressed either by a solid or liquid body. . . .
>
> These varying results depend on the greater or lesser diminution of the volume of air usually contained in the thorax (lungs); and the cause of which occasions this diminution, whether solid or liquid, produces analogous results to those obtained by striking a cask, for example, in different degrees of emptiness or fullness [Fig. 7–5]: the diminution of sound being proportioned to the diminution of the volume of air contained in it. . . .

Not content with these clinical observations, Auenbrugger sought experimental confirmation.

> The effect of effused fluids in producing the morbid sound, is at once proved by the injection of water into the thorax of a dead body; in which case it will be found that the sound elicited by percussion, will be obscure over the portion of the cavity occupied by the injected liquid.

The *technique* of percussion of the thorax requires both of the examiner's hands. The middle finger of the left hand is applied firmly interspace by interspace with the palm and other fingers lifted off the chest. The right middle finger of the free right hand is used to percuss the distal phalanx of the left finger applied to the chest wall using a *motion originating at the wrist.*

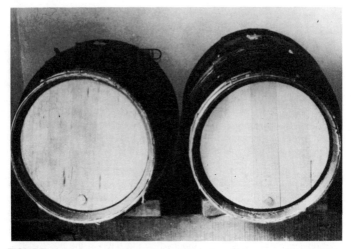

FIGURE 7–5. Burgundian wine casks. Auenbrugger witnessed his father's practice of percussing wine barrels to determine the level of their fluid content.

Two prime purposes of percussion of the thorax in the cardiac patient are to determine the presence, degree, and location (right versus left) of pleural effusions, and to determine the relative heights and movements of the hemidiaphragms. Diaphragmatic movement is assessed with the patient sitting. "When operating on the back, you are to cause the patient to bend forward, and draw his shoulder towards the anterior parts of the chest, so as to render the dorsal region rounded. . . ."[5] The bases of the right and left lungs are then percussed during full held inspiration and full held expiration, the difference in levels representing the excursion of the relevant hemidiaphragm. Hyperinflation of the lungs, as in pulmonary emphysema (see Fig. 7–3), is associated with reduced if not absent movement of the diaphragm.

The second role of percussion in cardiac patients is to seek out pleural effusions. "When water is collected in the cavity of the chest, between the pleura (costalis) and the lungs, the disease is called dropsy of the chest; and this is said to be of two kinds, namely, according as the fluid occupies one, or both sides. This is ascertained by percussion in the living subject; and is demonstrated by anatomical examination after death."[5] In congestive heart failure, pleural effusions are typically bilateral or isolated to the right, but are seldom isolated to the left.

An interesting variation on the theme of percussion is a patch of dullness beneath the angle of the left scapula. William Ewart described this sign in 1896 as evidence of a large *pericardial* effusion compressing the base of the left lung.[6] The eponym "Ewart's sign" is still used.

Auscultation of the human thorax was known to Hippocrates around 400 B.C.—the hippocratic succussion splash of hydropneumothorax.[7] Auscultation of the thorax in cardiac disease focuses on (1) abnormal diminution of the soft, low-pitched vesicular breath sounds heard during inspiration, (2) rales, (3) tubular breathing, (4) egophony, and (5) bronchophony, whispered pectoriloquy, wheezes, and pleural rubs.

Normal inspiratory vesicular breath sounds are reduced or absent in the hyperinflated lung of pulmonary emphysema (see Fig. 7–3), which often coexists with elevated pulmonary arterial pressure. Vesicular breath sounds are also reduced or absent in obesity (see Fig. 7–2).

Chest configuration and body build influence audibility of certain rales. In Richard C. Cabot's *Physical Diagnosis* (1915), rales are classified as (1) bubbling or nonconsonating, (2) crackling or consonating (the smallest varieties of this type are known as "crepitant" or "subcrepitant" rales, and (3) musical rales (squeaks or groans).[8] There is a current preference for grouping rales under the general category of "adventitious sounds." For the sake of historical continuity, I advise retaining the term *rale*, provided that what is heard is accurately described. Left ventricular failure is often associated with fine, crepitant, early and late inspiratory rales. These rales or crackles are produced by fluid in distal airways and alveoli. Coarser crackles originate in larger proximal airways.

Tubular breathing is often heard above a pleural effusion when the effusion causes compression atelectasis (consolidation). Additional auscultatory signs of consolidation take the form of egophony, bronchophony, and whispered pectoriloquy. Egophony is elicited by asking the patient to repeat "e, e, e," which is heard by the examiner as "a, a, a." It is the "e" to "a" change that is important. Whispered pectoriloquy represents amplification of the whispered "one-two-three" heard by the examiner over a zone of consolidation.

Wheezes are relatively pure, high-frequency musical acoustic events generated by air flow through narrowed bronchi. Wheezes are more likely to be heard during the expiratory effort, especially forced expiration. In pulmonary edema, the bronchial narrowing that is necessary for the generation of wheezes is caused by swelling and secretions. In emphysema, wheezes are caused by bronchospasm and mucus secretions.

Pleural rubs occur in patients with congestive heart failure chiefly because of pulmonary embolism with infarction. Hippocrates described the rub as "a sound like that made by leather. . . ."[7] Auscultation in search of rubs must be meticulous and conducted without haste. The patient should be made comfortable in a sitting position with the thorax relaxed and the elbows raised away from the chest wall. During normal breathing, the stethoscopic diaphragm is firmly applied over the lower lobes—axillae and back—because these are the common sites of pleural rubs caused by pulmonary infarction. The grating sound of the rub is typically heard during inspiration and expiration.

Thoracic auscultation occasionally detects what has been called the "cardiorespiratory murmur." Richard Cabot was aware that "cardiorespiratory murmurs may be produced without any adhesion of the lung to the pericardium under conditions not at present understood."[8] Cabot went on to say that:

> Such murmurs may be heard under the left clavicle or below the angle of the left scapula, as well as near the apex of the heart—less often in other parts of the chest. . . . Cardio-respiratory murmurs may be either systolic or diastolic, but the vast majority of cases are systolic. The area over which they are audible is usually a very limited one. They are greatly affected by position and by respiration, and are heard most distinctly if not exclusively during inspiration, especially at the end of that act.

Such murmurs were known to Laënnec, but the picturesque description of James Hope reinforces the image.[9] Hope described his experience with two university students:

> Both wore very tight waistcoats, preventing the expansion of the lower ribs. During this state of breathing, a bellows murmur . . . existed in both. In both, the murmur ceased entirely when, unbuttoning their waistcoats and waistbands of their trousers, they breathed with the lungs naturally inflated. By alternating the circumstances, the murmur could be created or removed at pleasure. I presume therefore that it proceeded from a cause exterior to the heart.

The mechanism responsible for the cardiorespiratory murmur remains unclear, but the location, timing, and relation to respiration remain as Cabot described.[8]

REFERENCES

1. Stokes, W.: Diseases of the Heart and Aorta. Dublin, Hodges and Smith, 1854.
2. Mackenzie, J.: Diseases of the Heart. London, Henry Frowde, 1908.
3. Burwell, C. S., Robin, E. D., Whaley, R. D., and Bicklemann, A. G.: Extreme obesity associated with alveolar hypoventilation—A pickwickian syndrome. Am. J. Med. 21:811, 1956.
4. Macklem, P. T., Macklem, D. M., and DeTroyer, A.: A model of respiratory muscle mechanics. J. Appl. Physiol. 55:547, 1983.
5. Auenbrugger, L.: On Percussion of the Chest. Vienna, 1761 (translated by John Forbes and published by T. and G. Underwood, London, 1824).
6. Ewart, W.: Practical aids in the diagnosis of pericardial effusion, in connection with the question as to surgical treatment. Brit. Med. J. March 21, 1896.
7. The Genuine Works of Hippocrates (translated from the Greek by Francis Adams). In Major, R. H.: Classic Descriptions of Disease. Springfield, Illinois, Charles C Thomas, Publisher, 1948.
8. Cabot, R. C.: Physical Diagnosis. New York, William Wood and Co., 1915.
9. Hope, J.: A Treatise on the Diseases of the Heart and Great Vessels. London, 1839.

THE ABDOMEN

Examination of the abdomen in the cardiac patient includes physical appearance (see Chapter 2), percussion, palpation, and auscultation. The flat supine position is preferable for assessment, with the abdomen exposed entirely. Once the patient is comfortable, the examination commences.

Physical appearance of the abdomen takes into account the normal and abnormal respiratory movements described in detail in Chapter 7. In the cardiac patient, protuberance of the abdomen arouses suspicion of ascites which, if tense, can cause eversion of the umbilicus. In a hypertensive patient, red to purple, depressed, lower abdominal striae suggest Cushing's syndrome as the cause of the hypertension.

Percussion establishes visceral situs by identifying gastric tympany on the left and hepatic dullness on the right in situs solitus (normal position) and the opposite in situs inversus (see Fig. 5–3). Although the percussion note is struck over the lower anterior thoracic cage, it is the abdominal viscera that are under scrutiny. Percussion of the liver proceeds from its upper border to its lower border, setting the stage for palpation (see below). While percussing gastric tympany in Traube's space, percussion can be extended just laterally in search of potential dullness from an enlarged spleen, heightening anticipation that the organ might be palpated (see below).

Percussion for detection of ascites requires special technique. With the patient supine and flat, fluid gravitates to the flanks, which are dull to percussion, while the lighter, air-filled intestines occupy the center of the abdomen in an area of relative tympany. Percussion identifies the line of demarcation from flank dullness to the tympanitic center. Once the line of demarcation has been established in the supine position, *shifting dullness* should be sought as the patient turns into a partial lateral decubitus position while the examiner again determines the dull-to-tympanitic line of demarcation. Ascites causes the demarcation to "shift" medially as the patient turns to the side—shifting dullness. With the patient again in the flat supine position, a fluid wave can be sought. The patient assists by compressing the center of the abdomen with the ulnar surface of either hand, while the examiner palpates one flank and taps the other. Detection of a fluid wave by the palpating hand suggests ascites unless the patient is obese or the ascitic volume is too small to transmit the fluid wave.

Palpation of the abdomen in the cardiac patient deals chiefly with the liver, spleen, abdominal aorta, and kidneys. Before attempting to palpate the liver edge, it is useful to estimate its upper and lower margins by percussion as described above. The palm of the examiner's right hand is then placed below the expected inferior hepatic margin lateral to the rectus muscle, while the left hand is placed posteriorly (Fig. 8–1). Flexion of the patient's knees or placing a pillow under the knees serves to relax the anterior abdominal wall and to improve the facility of palpation. The patient is asked to inhale slowly but deeply as the examiner presses the fingertips of the right hand upward and irward, anticipating the descent of the liver edge during inspiration. Care should be taken to palpate gently, because the liver is often tender in congestive hepatomegaly. The liver edge should be assessed for its consistency, its transverse extent (right/left), and its level below the right costal margin during full inspiration. In addition, careful palpation of the margin of the liver during a partially held inspiration permits detection of transmitted pulsations from the right atrium via the inferior cava (Fig. 8–2).

In infants, the breathing pattern does lend itself to selective palpation during inspiration, and the edge of

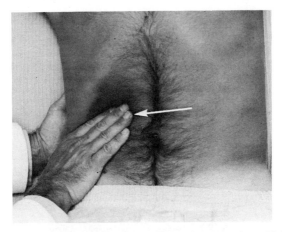

FIGURE 8–1. Palpation of the liver. The patient is supine with knees flexed to relax the abdomen. The flat of the examiner's right hand *(arrow)* is placed on the right upper quadrant just below the expected inferior margin of the liver; the left hand is applied diametrically opposite.

the congested liver is usually rounded and less distinct. Palpation commences once the infant is quiet (Fig. 8–3). The examiner should place the hand gradually and gently upon the abdomen so the infant becomes used to the contact. The right thumb is then applied to the right upper quadrant (right lobe) while the index finger palpates the left upper quadrant for the spleen. The right lobe of the liver is more readily palpable than the left. In an infant *without* congestive hepatomegaly, a transverse liver edge—extending from the right upper quadrant into the epigastrium—is an important physical sign of the visceral heterotaxy of asplenia or polysplenia in which there is a tendency for the liver to be bilaterally symmetric.[2]

Palpation of the *spleen* is somewhat more difficult than palpation of the liver and, in adults, requires examination in both the supine and right lateral decubitus positions. It is useful to begin by percussing lateral to the area of gastric tympany in the left upper quadrant (see above). Dullness in this area heightens suspicion of splenomegaly. The bed or examining table should be horizontal and

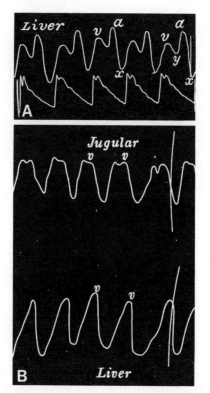

FIGURE 8–2. *A*, Simultaneous tracings of the liver pulse and the radial arterial pulse from Mackenzie.[1] The right atrial wave form is reflected in the liver pulse as the "A" wave, "X" descent, "V" wave, and "Y" descent. *B*, This figure, also from Mackenzie,[1] shows "the venous and liver pulses of the ventricular type" in a patient with tricuspid regurgitation. The "V" waves are tall, and the "Y" descents brisk if not collapsing.

the patient initially supine with the physician on the right at a level that permits the examiner's right hand to be applied to the patient's abdomen *without* flexing the wrist, thus avoiding a reduction in sensitivity of the fingertips. This is best achieved by having the examiner sit at the bedside or stand when the bed is higher or when an examining table is used. The palm of the examiner's right hand is placed below the left costal margin

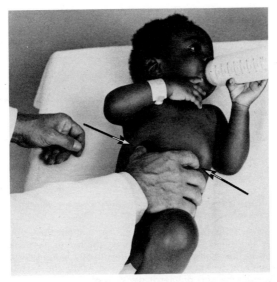

FIGURE 8–3. Palpation of liver and spleen in an infant. The thumb is applied to the right upper quadrant *(arrow)* while the index finger palpates the left upper quadrant *(second arrow)*. Separate attention should be paid to each organ, gently altering pressure first with the thumb, then with the finger as the infant breathes naturally and the liver and spleen descend during inspiration.

and pressed inward and upward toward the left shoulder, while the left hand is applied to the left posterior thorax to displace the spleen forward. The patient is then instructed to take a slow deep breath while the examiner palpates with the fingertips of the right hand, anticipating descent of the spleen during inspiration. If the spleen is not palpated convincingly in the supine position, palpation should be repeated in the right lateral decubitus (Fig. 8–4), a position that moves the spleen downward and anteriorly. The examiner places the right hand beneath the left costal margin and the left hand behind the posterior thorax, as shown in Figure 8–4. Note that the examiner's right wrist is not flexed, improving sensitivity of the fingertips as the patient takes a deep breath and the spleen descends. These maneuvers should be repeated

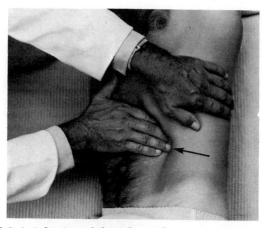

FIGURE 8–4. Palpation of the spleen. The patient turns toward the examiner so the left flank is raised above the bed or examining table. The palm of the examiner's right hand *(arrow)* is applied to the left upper quadrant without bending the wrist, while the examiner's left hand provides support diametrically opposite.

several times while readjusting the patient's tilt from the horizontal and the position of the palpating right hand in order to achieve optimal tactile sensitivity. A palpable spleen tip is often a subtle physical sign that requires diligence and practice to elicit with confidence. The principal settings in which splenomegaly is anticipated in cardiac patients are congestive enlargement and infective endocarditis. It is well to remember that in infective endocarditis the spleen is likely to be soft and tender, features that call for gentle palpation. In infants, palpation of the spleen is best achieved with the patient lying flat as the examiner applies the index finger of the right hand to the infant's left upper quadrant, as shown in Figure 8–3. Remember that the spleen tip is often palpable in normal newborns.

Abdominal aortic palpation should be routine and meticulous in older adults, especially the relatively high-risk older male with systemic hypertension. The patient should lie horizontal and supine with the anterior abdominal wall relaxed as described above for palpation of the liver. Partial flexion of the knees promotes relaxation, and a pillow beneath the patient's knees serves a useful purpose. The normal abdominal aorta is often palpable *above* the umbilicus, especially in multiparous women with relatively flaccid abdominal walls. The aorta is *not* normally palpable below the umbilicus. The examiner's right hand is first applied gently but firmly with gradually increasing pressure in the epigastrium *above* the umbilicus, recalling that the normal abdominal aorta can be tender. More important, however, is palpation of the abdominal aorta *inferior* to the umbilicus and to the left of midline. Routine palpation in this area is obligatory in relatively high-risk populations if asymptomatic abdominal aortic aneurysms are not to be overlooked. The patient should be instructed to breathe as quietly as possible, using thoracic respiratory muscles in order to minimize an inspiratory increase in abdominal girth. The fingertips of the examiner's right hand are then applied just below the umbilicus to the left of center. Pressure of the fingertips is gently and gradually increased in search of the aortic pulsation. While seeking the lateral margin of an abdominal aortic aneurysm, the palpating right hand should not only be applied with gradual and graded pressure, but should also attempt to "roll" the edge of the enlarged aorta under the fingertips. Once the lateral aortic margin is identified, bimanual palpation along the left and right margins of the aneurysm permits an experienced observer to estimate the size of the aneurysm. Size can be assessed by observing systolic separation of the index fingers placed on either side of the pulsating aorta. Remember that an enlarged or an enlarging abdominal aortic aneurysm is apt to be tender if not painful and, when leaking, causes pain in the low back (retroperitoneal) or in the posterior aspect of the left flank.

Palpation of the *kidneys* should be routine in adults and is obligatory in hypertensive adults. The technique is bimanual and performed with the patient supine and horizontal. For palpation of the right kidney, the examiner applies the palm of the right hand to the right upper quadrant with the tips of the fingers just below the costal margin. The left hand is placed behind the patient's flank diametrically opposite. The patient is instructed to take a gradual deep breath while the examiner's fingertips anticipate the descent of the lower pole of the kidney as a smooth rounded edge. Because the right kidney is lower than the left, its lower pole is occasionally palpable in normal persons. In palpating the *left* kidney, care should be taken to distinguish its lower pole from a palpable spleen. The technique for palpating the left kidney is similar to that just described, with the examiner's right hand applied to the patient's left upper quadrant with fingertips just beneath the left costal margin. The left hand is applied diametrically opposite on the left flank. In palpating either the right or left kidney, the examiner's hands should be approximated *while* the patient inhales deeply, but if the hands are brought together *before* inspiration, the kidney cannot descend and therefore may not be palpable. It is also well to recall that these techniques sometimes permit palpation of the kidney by either the *posterior* or *anterior* hand of the examiner. The most readily palpable kidneys are polycystic and must be palpated gently because of their delicate, cystic surfaces. Huge polycystic kidneys are large enough to be seen through the abdominal wall.

Auscultation is the final part of the abdominal examination. In the setting of cardiovascular disease, the stethoscope is used to seek abdominal aortic and iliofemoral systolic murmurs. With the patient supine, the diaphragm of the stethoscope is gently but firmly applied over the abdominal aorta beginning in the epigastrium and extending inferiorly below the umbilicus, to the right and left of midline, and then toward both the left and right inguinal ligaments along the courses of the iliac arteries. The degree of pressure of the stethoscope is adjusted to achieve maximal access to the abdominal aortic wall and its bifurcation. In the inguinal areas, the bell of the stethoscope is more practical than the diaphragm.

Renal arterial murmurs are infrequently detected, but should be routinely sought in hypertensive adults. Renal arterial auscultation begins with the patient sitting and the trunk relaxed to minimize interference from noise of tense muscles. The stethoscopic diaphragm is placed

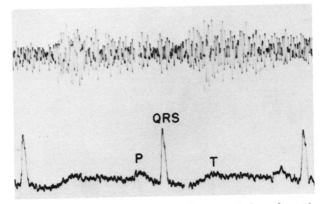

FIGURE 8–5. The continuous murmur of a congenital renal arteriovenous fistula in a 50-year-old woman whose systemic arterial blood pressure was within normal range. The murmur was best heard in the flank.

firmly against the skin of the posterior flank, first over one kidney and then over the other. The examination must be conducted in a room of absolute quiet, because renal arterial murmurs are, as a rule, soft and high-frequency. The patient is then re-examined in the supine position, with auscultation carried out by applying the diaphragm of the stethoscope anteriorly at the level appropriate for each renal artery just to the right and left of the abdominal aorta. High-frequency systolic murmurs occur with renal arterial stenosis. Rarely, the continuous murmur of a renal arteriovenous fistula is detected as the cause of systemic hypertension (Fig. 8–5).

REFERENCES

1. Mackenzie, J.: The Study of the Pulse, Arterial, Venous and Hepatic, and of the Movements of the Heart. Edinburgh, Young J. Pentland, 1902.
2. Perloff, J. K.: The Clinical Recognition of Congenital Heart Disease. 3rd ed. Philadelphia, W. B. Saunders Company, 1987.

INDEX

Page numbers in *italics* indicate illustrations; page numbers followed by (t) refer to tables.

271